Student Workbook to Accompany Sports Medicine Essentials, Core Concepts in Athletic Training & Fitness Instruction, 2nd Edition

Jim Clover, MEd, ATC, PTA

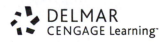

DELMAR
CENGAGE Learning

Australia • Brazil • Japan • Korea • Mexico • Singapore • Spain • United Kingdom • United States

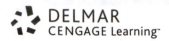
DELMAR
CENGAGE Learning™

Student Workbook to Accompany:
Sports Medicine Essentials, Core Concepts
in Athletic Training & Fitness Instruction,
Second Edition
Jim Clover

Vice President, Health Care Business Unit:
William Brottmiller

Director of Learning Solutions: Matthew Kane

Managing Editor: Marah Bellegarde

Acquisitions Editor: Matthew Seeley

Marketing Director: Jennifer McAvey

Marketing Channel Manager: Michele McTighe

Technology Director: Laurie Davis

Technology Project Coordinator: Carolyn Fox

Production Director: Carolyn Miller

Content Project Manager: Kenneth McGrath

For product information and technology assistance, contact us at
Cengage Learning Customer & Sales Support, 1-800-354-9706
For permission to use material from this text or product,
submit all requests online at **www.cengage.com/permissions**
Further permissions questions can be emailed to
permissionrequest@cengage.com

ExamView® and ExamView Pro® are registered trademarks of FSCreations, Inc. Windows is a registered trademark of the Microsoft Corporation used herein under license. Macintosh and Power Macintosh are registered trademarks of Apple Computer, Inc. Used herein under license.

Library of Congress Control Number: 2007010385

ISBN-13: 978-1-4018-6186-5

ISBN-10: 1-4018-6186-5

Delmar
Executive Woods
5 Maxwell Drive
Clifton Park, NY 12065
USA

Cengage Learning is a leading provider of customized learning solutions with office locations around the globe, including Singapore, the United Kingdom, Australia, Mexico, Brazil, and Japan. Locate your local office at **www.cengage.com/global**

Cengage Learning products are represented in Canada by Nelson Education, Ltd.

To learn more about Delmar, visit **www.cengage.com/delmar**

Purchase any of our products at your local bookstore or at our preferred online store **www.cengagebrain.com**

Notice to the Reader

Printed in the United States of America
3 4 5 6 7   14 13 12 11 10

ED308

Contents

Chapter 1: Careers in Sports Medicine

Assignment Sheet

Grade _____   Name _____

INTRODUCTION

You may follow any of a variety of pathways with the information you acquire in this text. After reading this chapter you will be able to understand which profession is best for you.

COMPLETION

1. What are the two careers listed in Chapter One?

    a.

    b.

2. What additional career possibilities could you establish based on the information in this book? Circle them in the following list.

    - sales of health-care supplies and services
    - family physician
    - orthopedic surgeon
    - strength and conditioning specialist
    - schoolteacher
    - nutritionist
    - physical therapy aide
    - certified athletic trainer
    - coach
    - physical therapist
    - personal trainer
    - sports medicine administrator
    - chiropractor
    - chiropractic aide
    - first aid provider
    - physician assistant
    - physical therapy assistant
    - entrepreneur in the health-care industry
    - retail sales of sporting goods
    - retail sales in a health-care supply store
    - strength coach
    - health club sales and marketing

3. What kind of person would be good in sports-medicine–related fields?

    a. They would have these traits:

b. Which traits do you have? (circle them). For the other traits (the ones you don't have), write next to the words, below, how you expect to deal with not having them.

4. Write your story about how you will get from here to your perfect job. Don't leave out any steps. Example: *I would like to work at Jim's Gym on the corner of 14th and Magnolia. To do that I will have to finish this course, get some letters of recommendation, fill out a job application, sit for an interview, understand the pay, and enjoy the hours I will be working.*

MATCHING

Match each item below to a statement or sentence listed on the right.

_____ 1. A branch of medicine that deals with the prevention and treatment of sports injuries

_____ 2. A discipline for someone who works in sports medicine

_____ 3. The person who combines knowledge and hands-on skill to increase athletes' safety

_____ 4. The use of heat, cold, or electrical stimulation to increase or decrease blood flow

_____ 5. BOC

_____ 6. A division of the sports medicine team that evaluates existing fitness levels

_____ 7. A characteristic needed for a position in sports medicine

_____ 8. NSCA

_____ 9. Sensitivity

_____ 10. Exercises designed to prepare an individual to become fit

a. Physical fitness program

b. Good listening skills

c. Sports medicine

d. Nutrition

e. Certified athletic trainer

f. Therapeutic modality

g. Certifying organization for the athletic trainer

h. Compassion

i. Strength and conditioning specialist

j. National Strength and Conditioning Association

TRUE/FALSE

_____ 1. Sports medicine is the study of the inactive population.

_____ 2. The certified athletic trainer is not a part of the sports medicine team.

____ 3. Therapeutic modalities are the use of heat or cold to increase or decrease blood flow.

____ 4. Fitness instructors help individuals improve their health.

____ 5. Communication skills are needed when dealing with athletes in pain.

____ 6. If you are going to tell someone to be fit, it would help if you were fit also.

____ 7. Leadership skills are for other people, not for those in sports medicine.

____ 8. Listening to athletes is very important in sports medicine.

____ 9. Once you pass this class, your education in sports medicine is complete.

____ 10. Your positive attitude will help improve athletes' attitudes.

SHORT ANSWER

1.   What classes will you need to take to get into the field of sports medicine?

2.   What fields of sports medicine interest you the most, and why?

3.   What would you have to do to become a certified athletic trainer?

4.   It is your first day on the job as a volunteer or intern athletic trainer at a local high school. What can you do right away to help the athletic trainer who is there?

Chapter 2: Athletic Training

Assignment Sheet

Grade _____   Name _____

INTRODUCTION

The athletic training career consists of the prevention and treatment of athletic injuries. The athletic trainer, once certified, can work with physically active people in many settings. These settings may vary from state to state, depending on state licensing laws. After you finish this chapter, you will have a better understanding of the field of athletic training.

COMPLETION

What are the job settings in which an athletic trainer might work?

a.

b.

c.

d.

e.

f.

g.

h.

i.

j.

k.

l.

m.

n.

o.

p.

MATCHING

Match each item below to a statement or sentence on the right.

_____ 1. The captain of the sports medicine team

_____ 2. The sports medicine team is partially composed of these

_____ 3. A professional skilled in the prevention, evaluation, treatment, and rehabilitation of sports injuries

_____ 4. Helps prevent further injuries to athletes by not letting them return to play before they are ready

_____ 5. Is responsible for making sure each athletic event and practice has someone who can provide proper first aid and CPR

_____ 6. EMS

_____ 7. Assumption of risk

_____ 8. Liability

_____ 9. Negligence

_____ 10. Pre-participation physical evaluation

a. Athletic trainer

b. The coach

c. The school administrator

d. Athletic trainer, physician, physical therapist, athlete, parents, and coach

e. Team physician

f. The failure to provide reasonable care

g. The form used prior to sports participation to find any preexisting injuries or illnesses

h. Legal responsibility

i. Individual assumes the responsibility he or she may get injured in the sport

j. Emergency Medical Services

TRUE/FALSE

_____ 1. The special instruction sheet is used for knowing what type of shoe is best for participation in a sport.

_____ 2. The athletic training student needs little, if any, supervision.

_____ 3. Preseason begins six to eight weeks before the season.

_____ 4. Intensity is how many times you work out per week.

_____ 5. The goal of an in-season conditioning program is to keep athletes from deconditioning during the season.

_____ 6. The athlete has primary responsibility to keep both the coach and athletic trainer aware of treatment history.

_____ 7. No conditioning program can ever prevent injuries.

_____ 8. The Emergency Insurance Information and Consent form is needed only at home athletic events.

_____ 9. Athletic training students can keep athletes hydrated during practice and games.

_____ 10. One of the athletic trainer's jobs is to prepare the playing field by setting up a water and first aid area.

_____ 11. HIPAA is a special certification for the certified athletic trainer.

_____ 12. The athletic trainer keeps records of all injuries of all persons who receive training.

SHORT ANSWER

1. Name three forms that must be completed before a student athlete may participate in a sports program.

2. Name two pre-existing illnesses for a student athlete that could cause stresses during athletic activities.

3. Name five foundational courses that an athletic training student must complete.

WORD SEARCH

Find the words that relate to athletic training in the following word-search grid.

```
U  Q  M  C  D  D  B  U  I  D  M  O  V  X  P  K  G  L  C  U  H  C  A  L  K
R  Z  E  N  A  E  P  N  E  F  I  L  I  V  V  O  V  M  P  H  Q  X  C  I  S
O  P  U  G  D  L  T  E  M  M  E  A  N  P  U  V  S  C  M  K  K  G  P  A  I
Q  K  P  V  G  E  O  I  Q  Q  O  W  T  U  O  A  F  T  X  H  E  Y  G  B  R
W  T  O  Q  N  A  N  R  J  Q  S  Z  F  S  H  O  M  S  S  T  Q  I  O  I  F
M  V  Q  S  A  O  H  C  I  X  J  W  T  B  R  T  J  Q  S  E  D  J  D  L  O
T  Q  I  H  R  O  G  Y  M  E  Y  K  C  I  P  I  A  Q  X  R  A  Y  S  I  N
F  T  E  S  A  R  W  X  D  V  S  M  D  J  K  W  F  W  Y  Y  B  S  D  T  O
Y  P  Q  Z  T  D  G  V  O  V  E  R  T  R  A  I  N  I  N  G  D  I  O  Y  I
E  M  E  R  G  E  N  C  Y  M  E  D  I  C  A  L  S  E  R  V  I  C  E  N  T
C  K  K  T  F  A  A  X  O  A  B  S  O  Y  S  P  N  A  I  C  I  S  Y  H  P
X  E  A  T  H  L  E  T  I  C  T  R  A  I  N  I  N  G  S  T  U  D  E  N  T
A  E  K  J  K  O  A  Q  N  N  U  S  Q  K  I  I  C  S  V  O  E  F  D  I  S
R  E  N  I  A  R  T  C  I  T  E  L  H  T  A  D  E  I  F  I  T  R  E  C  S
Z  R  B  E  Y  K  H  G  K  U  L  S  A  W  H  M  W  S  H  H  A  M  D  M  A
H  C  A  O  C  S  L  R  I  P  L  R  G  P  Z  U  A  A  X  U  R  T  V  T  N
B  S  Z  Q  U  T  E  O  F  K  U  S  T  R  E  N  G  T  H  Z  D  Q  W  Y  D
K  C  S  M  H  U  T  Y  E  D  G  B  A  P  M  J  I  A  G  X  Y  I  T  F  Y
T  C  N  Y  D  B  E  S  M  O  V  K  P  U  V  R  I  I  Y  D  H  R  E  Y  X
```

ASSUMPTION OF RISK
CERTIFIED ATHLETIC TRAINER
EMERGENCY MEDICAL SERVICE
INTENSITY
NATA
POSTSEASON

ATHLETE
COACH
FIRST AID
LIABILITY
OVERTRAINING
STRENGTH

CALORIES
DURATION
HYDRATED
MINORS
PHYSICIAN
ATHLETIC TRAINING STUDENT

Chapter 3: Strength and Conditioning Specialist

Assignment Sheet

Grade _____   Name _____

INTRODUCTION

With health and fitness fads always coming and going, the strength and conditioning specialist must have the proper educational foundation to know what is real and what is not. This chapter will provide that information.

If you "channel surf" through multiple television channels, you will see an array of different fads for getting fit and losing weight. In the space below, write down the ones you've seen recently (and we'll see which ones last the length of this course!).

Whether you win or lose in promoting fitness will be mostly up to you. Your appearance, excitement, imagination, and knowledge will make or break you. You have to establish and separate yourself from the rest.

COMPLETION/SHORT ANSWER

1. Get a copy of your local yellow pages or search them online. What fitness-related jobs or workplaces, if any, are listed there?

2. What fitness jobs or settings that you know about are *not* available in your community?

3. What are some skills and personal traits that you like in a person? Which of those do you currently have but would like to improve?

4. Create a personal fitness program for yourself. Fill in the name, goal, and beginning portions of the Goal Review Record. Keep track of your progress on the Fitness Progress Record. Come back to the Goal Review Record weekly and chart your progress toward your personal fitness goal.

Goal Review Record

Name:	Personal Goal:			
	Weight	**% Body Fat**	**Sit-ups**	**[Other]**
Date: Beginning				
Date: Review 1				
Date: Review 2				
Date: Review 3				
Date: Final				

Fitness Progress Record

Name:	Fitness Progress			
Date:	Exercise	Duration/Sets	Repetitions	Weight

5. Interview one adult and one person your age and ask them about fitness. Then answer the following questions for each interviewee.

   a. Have they ever started a fitness program?

   b. If so, what did they like about it, and why did they stick with it or stop it?

   c. If they have never participated in a fitness program, why not? What it would take for them to participate in a fitness program?

MATCHING

Match each item below to a statement or sentence listed on the right.

_____ 1. Physical fitness

_____ 2. Multitasking skills

_____ 3. Physical fitness fads

_____ 4. SCS

_____ 5. Advance contact

_____ 6. Rapport

_____ 7. Strength

_____ 8. Active listening

_____ 9. Objective evaluation

_____ 10. Subjective evaluation

_____ 11. Flexibility

_____ 12. Muscle endurance

_____ 13. ROM

_____ 14. Body composition

_____ 15. Positive verbal cue

a. Trendy diets, complicated exercise equipment

b. Nodding your head and responding verbally to your client

c. Good relationships and communication with clients

d. The strength, endurance, and mental well-being to be comfortable in daily, recreational, and sports activities

e. Based on the client's perception

f. Amounts of water, fat tissue, and lean tissue

g. Words that encourage and reinforce the client's efforts

h. The ability to stretch a muscle through the full ROM

i. Sending a reminder or calling ahead of scheduled time of session

j. Muscle's ability to exert a maximum force against resistance

k. Range of motion

l. Skills that enable a person to competently perform more than one task at a time

m. Strength and conditioning specialist

n. Muscle's ability to apply repeated force over a period of time

o. Measurements based on facts

TRUE/FALSE

_____ 1. Music should not be used as a motivational tool for a client.

_____ 2. Your appearance and the appearance of the establishment in which you work are very important.

_____ 3. You should always trust the information in the latest fitness trends.

_____ 4. Goals should be put in writing.

_____ 5. As a strength and conditioning specialist it is important that you know your client's physical limitations.

_____ 6. When establishing a client's fitness profile, knowing the client's body composition is not important.

_____ 7. Objective evaluation is not based on measurable facts.

_____ 8. It is acceptable to be late for your appointments.

_____ 9. ACSM stands for American College of Sports Medicine.

_____ 10. A strength and conditioning specialist is a person with the knowledge, skills, and motivation to enhance the physical fitness of individuals.

CROSSWORD PUZZLE

Use the clues to complete this strength and conditioning specialist crossword puzzle.

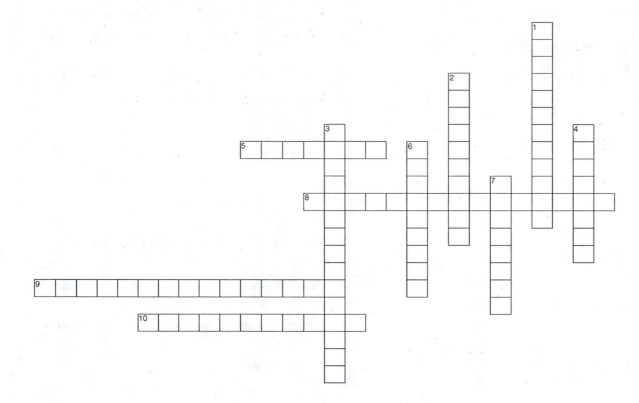

Across

5. Establishing and maintaining good relationships and communication with clients
8. When your client is talking to you, and you nod your head in response, and respond verbally to your client's concerns
9. The strength, endurance, and mental well-being to be comfortable in daily activities
10. Ability to stretch a muscle through its full range of motion without causing pain or muscle tearing

Down

1. Skills that enable a person to competently perform more than one task at a time
2. Based on your client's perception
3. Ratio between lean body mass and fat
4. It is important to _____ your client's records
6. Based on measurable facts
7. Ability of a muscle to exert a maximum force against a resistance

Chapter 4: Ethical and Legal Considerations

Assignment Sheet

Grade _____   Name _____

INTRODUCTION

In becoming a professional in any vocation, you take on specific legal and ethical responsibilities. The reality of becoming an athletic trainer, personal trainer, or going into the field of physical therapy is that most things you do will be performed in a public area where many bystanders will have a view of (and opinion about) what you are doing. Because of this, you can be more susceptible to legal action. Remember that most lawsuits are initiated because of desire for financial gain, improper follow-through, or because someone was angered.

One of the ways to prevent lawsuits is to prepare written guidelines *before* you initiate care or establish an exercise program. Remember that you are venturing into areas that can produce injuries. Your job, as a professional, is to ensure that the best treatment and follow-through is available. To do this, you must be prepared with the proper education, supplies, and equipment in case an injury does occur.

COMPLETION/SHORT ANSWER

1. You are putting together a sports medicine team. Who might be some of the people involved? What would be their duties? Name the person and the duties the person would perform.

Person	Duties
a.	
b.	
c.	
d.	
e.	
f.	

2. What are the rules for scholastic eligibility for athletes at your school? Do you agree with them? If not, how would you change them?

3. Why is a written code of ethics important?

4. The legal responsibility for any loss or damage that occurs as a result of one or more person's action or inaction is called

5. A private or civil wrong against another person or that person's property is called

6. The failure to give reasonable care or to do what another prudent person with similar experience, knowledge, and background would have done under the same or similar circumstances is called

7. Risk management involves

8. What is a primary risk?

9. What is a secondary risk?

10. Fill in the second column below. The first letter of each word in the answers (*SAFE*) is in the first column.

S		Someone must be present to provide this from the locker room to the practice or event
A		Provide proper assistance when the athlete needs it
F		Must be checked daily for hazards
E		Must be checked daily for proper maintenance

11. Name three reasons a person might file a lawsuit.

   a.

   b.

   c.

12. Name and describe eight ways to make sports safer for athletes—and prevent lawsuits.

   a.

   b.

   c.

   d.

   e.

   f.

   g.

   h.

13. Bring the forms from your athletic team or department to class (e.g., code of ethics, standards of conduct, etc.). Discuss what is good about these forms and what needs to be improved.

MATCHING

Match each item below to a statement or sentence listed on the right.

_____ 1. Risk management

_____ 2. Negligence

_____ 3. Standard of care

_____ 4. Ethics

_____ 5. Litigation

_____ 6. Tort

_____ 7. Battery

_____ 8. Malpractice

_____ 9. Patient's Bill of Rights

_____ 10. A reason for litigation

_____ 11. Safety committee

a. Morals; a set of principles or values that influence behavior

b. Professional misconduct or lack of professional skill that results in injury to a patient

c. Private or civil wrong against another person or his or her property

d. Degree of care, skill, and diligence ordinarily exercised by other caregivers under the same or similar circumstances

e. Reduction of the potential for injury

f. The patient has the right to considerate and respectful care

g. Failure to give reasonable care

h. Sexual harassment

i. Unlawful touching of an individual without consent

j. Group of diverse individuals brought together to identify athletes' safety concerns

k. A lawsuit

TRUE/FALSE

_____ 1. The patient does not have the right to know what hospital rules and regulations apply to his or her conduct as a patient.

_____ 2. The patient has the right to obtain from the physician complete and current information about his or her diagnosis.

_____ 3. The patient has the right to expect that all communication and records pertaining to his or her care are treated as confidential.

_____ 4. The patient does not have the right to say no to being part of a research project.

_____ 5. The patient has the right to obtain information about the existence of any professional relationships among individuals that are treating him or her.

WORD SEARCH

Find and circle the words related to ethical and legal issues.

```
s  c  i  h  t  e  f  o  e  d  o  c  q  s  a
b  a  t  o  r  t  h  b  q  w  e  b  t  j  d
j  o  f  z  m  c  v  y  w  c  d  a  n  k  m
t  l  d  e  a  q  h  d  n  t  n  t  o  s  i
e  l  i  o  t  b  k  e  p  d  g  t  i  c  n
w  c  c  a  t  y  g  n  a  w  d  e  t  i  i
t  k  i  w  b  i  c  r  d  c  j  r  a  h  s
s  u  a  t  l  i  d  o  o  u  e  y  g  t  t
e  q  k  g  c  o  l  n  m  j  t  q  i  e  r
y  g  e  i  f  a  d  i  e  m  y  y  t  c  a
x  n  a  c  m  u  r  c  t  v  i  n  i  p  t
b  a  a  m  c  a  f  p  c  y  r  t  l  x  i
f  r  i  t  a  e  t  e  l  h  t  a  t  h  o
e  i  l  o  g  d  r  z  k  a  q  g  j  e  n
m  a  n  a  g  e  m  e  n  t  m  l  h  d  e
```

administration
athlete
battery
coach
code of ethics
conduct
damage
duty
ethics
liability
litigation
malpractice
management
negligence
safety committee
standard of care
tort

17

Chapter 5: Physical Fitness Assessment

Assignment Sheet

Grade _____   Name _____

INTRODUCTION

To be successful in the field of sports medicine, you must know how to assess fitness. You must be able to document where your clients fit—or do not fit—within the norms.

This chapter will give you the knowledge and skills to provide a physical assessment that establishes a baseline for clients from which to start their physical activity. Once you have this information, you can then offer goals and time frames to meet those goals.

COMPLETION/SHORT ANSWER

1. The strength, endurance, and mental well-being required to be competitive in a defined level of sports activity is called

2. The ability to perform daily activities with vitality and energy, to withstand stress without undue fatigue, and to maintain physical health without medical intervention is called

3. Use the following fitness evaluation to organize and track the different elements of fitness evaluation and see how you respond to each. Have a friend help keep count and an instructor supervise each element.

Name:		Date		Date			Comments
Fitness Evaluation	**#**	**Peer Check-off** Yes	No	**Instructor Check-off** Yes	No	**Points Earned**	
Bent-leg sit-ups (1 min)							
Push-ups/modified (to fatigue)							
Bench jump/step (1 min)							
Sit and reach (in.)							
Back bend (in.)							
Resting heart rate (bpm)							
Pulse recovery step test (bpm)							
Weight (lbs)							
Body fat							
Ideal weight							

4. The first table below shows how to determine ideal weight. Use the following three tables to determine your ideal weight and the ideal weights of two others.

Determine Ideal Weight (Example)

Body weight	145 lbs	
% Body fat	27%	
Body weight (145)	Times % B.F. (0.27)	Equals (39 lbs) of fat
Body weight (145)	Minus lbs of fat (39)	Equals (106 lbs) of lean body mass

Client One

Body weight	lbs	
% Body fat	%	
Body weight ( )	Times % B.F. (0.)	Equals (lbs) of fat
Body weight ( )	Minus lbs of fat ( )	Equals (lbs) of lean body mass

Client Two

Body weight	lbs	
% Body fat	%	
Body weight ( )	Times % B.F. (0.)	Equals (lbs) of fat
Body weight ( )	Minus lbs of fat ( )	Equals (lbs) of lean body mass

Client Three

Body weight	lbs	
% Body fat	%	
Body weight ( )	Times % B.F. (0.)	Equals (lbs) of fat
Body weight ( )	Minus lbs of fat ( )	Equals (lbs) of lean body mass

a. What are the percentage body-fat goals of

Client One?

Client Two?

Client Three?

b. How much weight will each client have to lose to reach that goal?

Client One?

Client Two?

Client Three?

5. Look at the "Physical Assessment Form" in Chapter 5 of your book.

a. What might be some of the warning signs that the fitness program may have to be altered to match physical limitations or restrictions?

b. What special equipment do you need, if any?

MATCHING

Match each item below to a statement or sentence listed on the right.

_____ 1. Competitive fitness

_____ 2. General fitness

_____ 3. Repetition

_____ 4. Contraction

_____ 5. Hamstrings

_____ 6. Resting heart rate

_____ 7. Recovery heart rate

_____ 8. Lean body weight

_____ 9. Fat weight

_____ 10. Essential body fat

_____ 11. Ideal percentage of body fat

_____ 12. Recommended body-fat percentage for a male less than age 30

_____ 13. Recommended body-fat percentage for a female less than age 30

_____ 14. Essential body fat for females

_____ 15. Multiply by this to know the number of pounds of fat a female has

a. Shortening or tightening of a muscle

b. Number of times the heart beats in 1 minute when no physical activity is taking place

c. Minimum amount of body fat necessary for the proper protection of the internal organs

d. 9–15%

e. Strength, endurance, and mental well-being required to be competitive in sports activities

f. Weight of the body after the fat weight has been subtracted

g. Total body weight by a woman's percentage of body fat

h. Completion of a designated movement through the entire range of motion

i. Muscles on the posterior aspect of the femur

j. Ability to perform daily activities with vitality and energy, to withstand stress without undue fatigue, and to maintain physical health without medical intervention

k. 14–21%

l. 11%

m. Amount of fat at which a person performs and feels her best

n. Number of times the heart beats in 1 minute, 60 seconds after completion of 3 minutes or more of exercise

o. Weight of the body after lean body weight has been subtracted

TRUE/FALSE

_____ 1. The sit-and-reach is a test for quadriceps flexibility.

_____ 2. A good test to determine muscle endurance of the lower extremities is the bench jump.

_____ 3. The push-up tells how much you can squat with your legs.

_____ 4. A high fitness level for abdominal muscle endurance, for a female age 35, would be the ability to do 39 bent-leg sit-ups in 1 minute.

_____ 5. A medium fitness level for upper-body muscle endurance, for a male age 35, would be 16 push-ups to fatigue.

_____ 6. An above-average score for flexibility in a woman at the age of 57 would be 17.

_____ 7. Recommended body-fat percentage for a male age 55 would be 24%.

_____ 8. The average systolic pressure is 65–90 mm Hg.

_____ 9. Skinfold calipers are calibrated in inches.

_____ 10. Because physical and medical conditions are not always readily apparent, all individuals should see a physician and be cleared for participation in strenuous activity before beginning a training program.

WORD SEARCH

Find the words related to physical fitness assessment.

```
k c e l k s h e z w i y l m r r l n a k
q c o c u u e l d v u o e y e f d c j o
s s e n t i f e v i t i t e p m o c l m
e n m z t k c e h h n z g b e g w o i f
y t u s n r c m a y a b g y t s l e a t
t g a u d e a m x g y n y s i p j t k y
l h r r b s c j z u z s h t u m a v m
i t g h t t x b t i f e o x i h m r a s
e u x i r r p w v i n q f w o s p t l w
c u o i e x a d f t o t a y n u o r j i
y i n i b w c e i x p n l r g p t a s v
j g a j r k t f h f y q v i q t w e z n
s t f m w s l a x y v n p s g c r h j s
r i m v l a x b f c r f z c p y f g m n
i r k e r j l a t i n e g n o c a n b d
x i v e h g d b t x p v v e n c l i k q
r m n r d n e h i y x z o o h b p t c c
l e a n b o d y w e i g h t c s k s l c
g z b d w d q v b e r d v w z e n e j p
c q w t p l t k d m u a d d c q r r k n
```

competitive fitness
congenital
contraction
fat weight
general fitness
hamstrings
lean body weight
push-ups
recovery heart rate
repetition
resting heart rate
trunk

Chapter 6: Nutrition and Weight Management

Assignment Sheet

Grade _____   Name _____

INTRODUCTION

People have a variety of eating plans, from getting up in the morning and grabbing a diet soda and a handful of candy to taking a shot of wheatgrass. Most nutrition plans are based on time limitations, accessibility to certain types of foods, how the food makes you feel, and sometimes even the right nutritional thing to do.

People are always looking for a quick fix, from what they see in the latest commercial to what a neighbor or friend told them. This, instead of understanding about nutrition, often determines what people eat. This chapter will provide you with nutritional facts. Then it will be your job to provide that knowledge to your clients.

COMPLETION/SHORT ANSWER

1. Go to the grocery store and find 15 items. Using the table below, write down their nutritional facts.

Item	Servings per Container	Calories	Calories from Fat	Total Fat	Cholesterol	Sodium	Sugar (grams)	Carbohydrates (grams)
.								

2. Go to four local fast-food restaurants and get their nutritional fact sheets. Once you have them, plan meals for five days, using the following tables.

Monday

Item	Servings per Container	Calories	Calories from Fat	Total Fat	Cholesterol	Sodium	Sugar (grams)	Carbohydrates (grams)
Breakfast								
Lunch								
Dinner								

Tuesday

Item	Servings per Container	Calories	Calories from Fat	Total Fat	Cholesterol	Sodium	Sugar (grams)	Carbohydrates (grams)
Breakfast								
Lunch								
Dinner								

Wednesday

Item	Servings per Container	Calories	Calories from Fat	Total Fat	Cholesterol	Sodium	Sugar (grams)	Carbohydrates (grams)
Breakfast								
Lunch								
Dinner								

Thursday

Item	Servings per Container	Calories	Calories from Fat	Total Fat	Cholesterol	Sodium	Sugar (grams)	Carbohydrates (grams)
Breakfast								
Lunch								
Dinner								

Friday

Item	Servings per Container	Calories	Calories from Fat	Total Fat	Cholesterol	Sodium	Sugar (grams)	Carbohydrates (grams)
Breakfast								
Lunch								
Dinner								

3. Now add up the calories you would have taken in each day.

Monday	
Tuesday	
Wednesday	
Thursday	
Friday	

4. If you would have taken in more calories than you should have, write down activities and the lengths of time you would have to participate in those activities to burn off the extra calories.

Activity	Length of Time	Calories Expended

5. If you would have taken in fewer calories than you should have, write down what additional food you can eat each day.

Monday	
Tuesday	
Wednesday	
Thursday	
Friday	

6. Describe a safe method to increase your weight.

7. Describe a safe method to decrease your weight.

8. Give an example of an appropriate pre-event meal.

9. What eating disorder is characterized by bingeing on large amounts of food followed by purging (vomiting)?

10. What eating disorder is characterized by refusal to eat a sufficient amount of food to maintain weight?

MATCHING

Match each item below to a statement or sentence listed on the right.

_____ 1. Metabolism

_____ 2. Nutrients

_____ 3. Carbohydrate

_____ 4. Glycogen

_____ 5. Calories

_____ 6. Protein

_____ 7. Fat

_____ 8. HDLs

_____ 9. Dietary fiber

_____ 10. Vitamins

_____ 11. Minerals

_____ 12. Dehydration

_____ 13. Dietary reference intakes

_____ 14. Food guide pyramid

_____ 15. Basal metabolic rate

a. Primary fuel needed by athletes in most sports

b. Substance made up of lipids or fatty acids that is a source of energy and is vital to growth and development

c. Roughage

d. Set of nutrient reference values used to plan and evaluate diets for good health

e. Sum of all physical and chemical processes that take place in the body; the conversion of food to energy

f. Unit of heat

g. Organic substances, other than proteins, carbohydrates, fats, and organic salts, that are essential in small quantities for normal bodily function

h. Substances that provide nourishment

i. Any of a class of complex, nitrogenous organic compounds that function as the primary building blocks of the body

j. High-density lipoproteins

k. Loss of water from a body or substance

l. Rate at which the body normally burns calories

m. General guide for healthy eating that illustrates the number of recommended daily servings for each food group and emphasizes a diet rich in variety

n. Organic compounds essential to bodily function

o. Complex sugar that is a basic source of energy for the body

TRUE/FALSE

_____ 1. The safe goal for gaining lean weight is 2 to 3 pounds per week.

_____ 2. Nutritional quacks are people who have the skills and knowledge they claim to have.

_____ 3. Advertisers claim that ergogenic aids enhance athletic performance.

_____ 4. A proper pre-exercise meal prevents hunger during exercise and helps maintain an adequate blood sugar level.

_____ 5. Eating sugar before exercise will help you run faster.

_____ 6. A high-carbohydrate diet (50–60% of calories consumed per day) will help speed recovery from physical exertion.

_____ 7. Anorexia nervosa is a disorder that usually begins in adolescence and is much more common in females than in males.

_____ 8. Bulimia nervosa is characterized by bingeing on large amounts of food, followed by inappropriate behavior, such as vomiting.

____ 9. Anorexia means a severe loss of appetite.

____ 10. Treatment for someone with bulimia does not include monitoring the person's eating.

CROSSWORD PUZZLE

Use the clues to complete this crossword puzzle about nutrition and weight management.

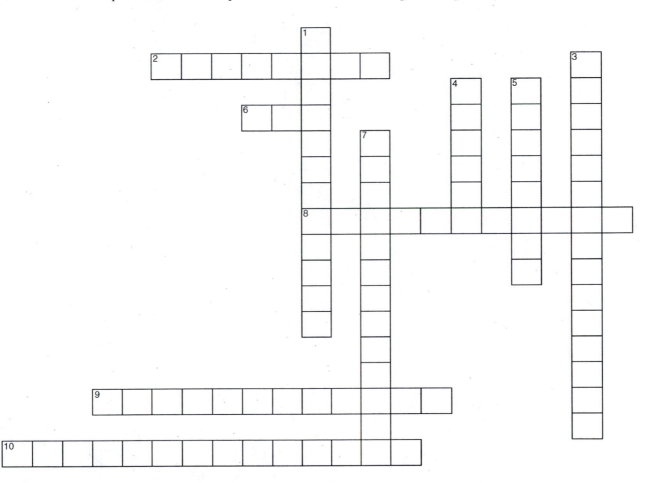

Across

2. Organic compounds that the body requires in small amounts but can manufacture
6. A substance made up of lipids or fatty acids that is a source of energy
8. Serves as an educational tool to put the dietary guidelines into practice
9. High sodium intake can contribute to _____ in sodium-sensitive individuals
10. Bingeing on large amounts of food, followed by inappropriate behavior

Down

1. The portion of plant foods that cannot be digested
3. Severe loss of appetite
4. The sum of the caloric content in food ingested is known as the _____ intake
5. Inorganic compounds
7. Represent one of the latest trends of sports nutrition

Chapter 7: Physical Conditioning

Assignment Sheet

Grade _____   Name _____

INTRODUCTION

There are several different ways to prepare the body for optimized performance. One of the goals of studying sports medicine is to learn exercises that are based on the client or athlete's goals. These goals for best performance are different than the goal of rehabilitation or the goal to increase strength. When you are finished with this chapter, you will have a better understanding of how to use flexibility exercises to reduce the risk of injury, and of how to safely guide clients and athletes through effective conditioning exercises.

MATCHING

Match each item below to a statement or sentence on the right.

_____ 1. Conditioning

_____ 2. Muscle tone

_____ 3. Power

_____ 4. Muscle mass

_____ 5. Overload principle

_____ 6. Variation principle

_____ 7. Specificity principle

_____ 8. Stretching

_____ 9. Resistance

_____ 10. Isometric contraction

_____ 11. Isotonic contraction

_____ 12. Isokinetic contraction

_____ 13. Set

a. Group of repetitions

b. Counterforce

c. Way in which an exercise relates to the activity for which performance enhancement is sought

d. Shape of a muscle in its resting state

e. Muscle contraction produced by a constant external resistance

f. Muscle contraction with no motion that results in no change in its resting state

g. Muscle contraction produced by a variable external resistance at a constant speed

h. Girth or size of a muscle

i. Application of greater-than-normal stress to a muscle, resulting in increased capacity to do work

j. Ability to apply force with speed

k. Process of preparing the body for optimized performance

l. Alteration or modification of exercises to work an entire muscle or group of muscles

m. Gently forcing the muscle to lengthen

SHORT ANSWER

1. Name the three basic principles of weight training, and briefly compare and contrast each.

   a.

   b.

   c.

2. Name the seven safety guidelines for weight training

   a.

   b.

   c.

   d.

   e.

   f.

   g.

COMPLETION

Flexibility Exercises for Target Areas

For each body part listed in the first column of the table, list its muscle groups and the stretching exercises for each muscle group.

Body Part	Muscle Group	Stretching Exercise
Neck		
Chest		
Shoulders		a. b.
Arms	a. b.	a. b.
Trunk/hips	a. b. c. d. e.	a. b. c. d. e.

Body Strengthening Exercises for Target Areas

For each body part listed in the first column of the table, list its muscle groups and the strengthening exercises for each muscle group.

Body Part	Muscle Group	Strengthening Exercise
Chest		a. b. c.
Shoulders		a. b. c.
Trunk/Hips	a. b. c. d. e. f.	a. b. c. d. e. f.
Legs	a. b. c.	a. b. c.

TRUE/FALSE

_____ 1. Muscle mass is the shape of a muscle in its resting state.

_____ 2. In starting a fitness program, it is not important to ensure the client is having fun.

_____ 3. The overload principle is the application of a greater-than-normal stress to a muscle.

_____ 4. The specificity principle refers to the relationship between having fun and the activity.

_____ 5. One way to avoid muscle cramping is to stay hydrated.

_____ 6. Isometric exercise is a contraction with no motion.

_____ 7. Isotonic exercise is the same weight through the range of motion.

_____ 8. Proprioception is the balance of time for an exercise.

_____ 9. The chest fly on a guided weight machine would be a good exercise to strengthen the chest muscles.

_____ 10. The seated row will help strengthen the lower legs.

_____ 11. If an offensive guard on the football team wanted to strengthen his quadriceps, he could do squats.

_____ 12. A client who wants to strengthen her upper body should use a UBE.

CROSSWORD PUZZLE

Use the clues to complete this crossword puzzle about physical conditioning.

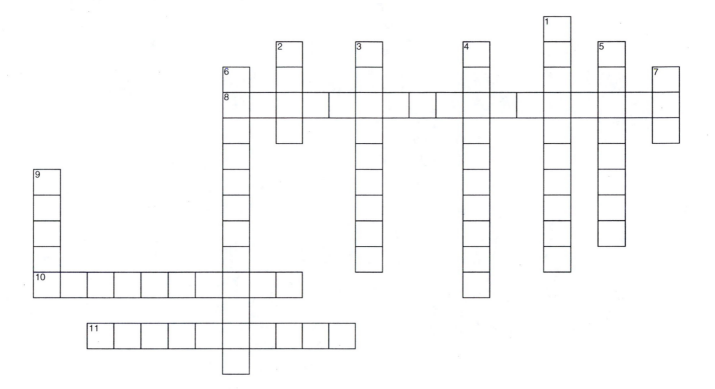

Across

8. Application of greater-than-normal stress to a muscle
10. Counterforce
11. A muscle contraction produced by a variable external resistance at a constant speed

Down

1. The girth or size of a muscle
2. A healthy _____ is vital to any conditioning program
3. A muscle contraction with no motion that results in no change in the length of the muscle
4. Gently forcing the muscle to lengthen
5. Maximum capability
6. Process of preparing the body for optimized performance
7. A group of repetitions is known as a _____
9. The ability to apply force with speed

Chapter 8: Designing a Conditioning Program

Assignment Sheet

Grade _____   Name _____

INTRODUCTION

There are several factors to consider when trying to build a successful fitness program. The program should have a foundation, a structure, and the ability to meet a client's needs. The foundation consists of the client's goals, time schedule, habits, and personal preferences. The structure consists of the mode, intensity, duration, frequency, special considerations, fun, and relaxation. Each of the preceding elements is vital to the success of a client's program. After reading this chapter, you will have a better understanding of how to design a successful conditioning program.

FILL IN THE BLANK

Complete these sentences using the following list of words (some words may be used more than once).

physician	subjective	mode	periodization
objective	target zone	frequency	intensity
injury	5 to 10 minutes	routine	duration
safety	needs		

1.   _____ is the first rule of conditioning, and a physician's clearance is the best way of ensuring that your clients get off to a good start.

2.   These goals should be written as _____, measurable goals, rather than subjective goals. _____ data is harder to measure and evaluate.

3.   Do not set goals so high that clients push themselves and risk _____. Help them build a _____ slowly, and show them how to warm up safely with stretching and _____ of cardiorespiratory exercise before the workout, and cool down slowly with _____ of flexibility exercises afterward.

4.   The _____ refers to the types of exercise and equipment you feel is most appropriate for your client to perform to accomplish her fitness goals.
     _____ is the degree of effort required to complete a physical activity.
     _____ refers to the length of time an activity is performed.
     _____ refers to the number of times something is done.

5.   A repeating schedule for exercise is also known as a _____.

6.   Year-round conditioning, known as _____, dictates that small amounts of work be added to each practice period as capacity increases.

7.   Regardless of whether you are doing individual or group instruction, you must always make sure that your clients or athletes have been cleared by a _____ before they begin a conditioning program.

8.   If you work with clients one-on-one, you will need to tailor each program to the client's _____.

MULTIPLE CHOICE

Circle the best answer.

1. The first rule of conditioning is
   a. physician's clearance
   b. know your client
   c. safety
   d. reviewing your client's health history

2. In designing a conditioning program, you should include
   a. intensity, duration, mode, and frequency
   b. intensity, target zone, duration, and mode
   c. mode, duration, intensity, and relaxation
   d. relaxation, fun, target zone, and duration

3. The rule that dictates that small amounts of work be added to each practice period as capacity increases is called
   a. periodization
   b. motivation
   c. modification
   d. progression

4. A subjective goal would be
   a. percentage of body fat
   b. weight
   c. how you feel
   d. waistline

5. What is a special population?
   a. people who are right-handed
   b. people with low back problems
   c. people with a size 12 shoe
   d. people who like to wake up early

PERSONAL WORKOUT

Now that you have read Chapter 8, use the following tables to put together a brief conditioning program for yourself. The program should include exercise mode, intensity, frequency, and duration.

Monday/Wednesday/Friday			
Cardiorespiratory Workout	Mode	Duration	Heart Rate
Arms (Biceps)	Mode	Repetitions	
Arms (Triceps)	Mode	Repetitions	
Chest	Mode	Repetitions	
Back	Mode	Repetitions	
Trunk	Mode	Repetitions	
Hamstrings	Mode	Repetitions	
Quadriceps	Mode	Repetitions	
Other	Mode	Repetitions	
Other	Mode	Repetitions	
Other	Mode	Repetitions	
Other	Mode	Repetitions	
Flexibility Exercises	Mode	Repetitions	
	Mode	Repetitions	
	Mode	Repetitions	
	Mode	Repetitions	
	Mode	Repetitions	
Game Activity (racquetball, etc.)			

Tuesday/Thursday			
Cardiorespiratory Workout	Mode	Duration	Heart Rate
Arms (Biceps)	Mode	Repetitions	
Arms (Triceps)	Mode	Repetitions	
Chest	Mode	Repetitions	
Back	Mode	Repetitions	
Trunk	Mode	Repetitions	
Hamstrings	Mode	Repetitions	
Quadriceps	Mode	Repetitions	
Other	Mode	Repetitions	
Other	Mode	Repetitions	
Other	Mode	Repetitions	
Other	Mode	Repetitions	
Flexibility Exercises	Mode	Repetitions	
	Mode	Repetitions	
	Mode	Repetitions	
	Mode	Repetitions	
	Mode	Repetitions	
Game Activity (racquetball, etc.)			

Time Schedule	
Goal	
Existing Habits and Preferences	
Fun	
Music	
Amount of Rest Needed	
Progression Expected	
Cardio Mode Variety	
Special Considerations	

TRUE/FALSE

_____ 1. Safety is the first rule of conditioning.

_____ 2. Goals do not help to determine the types of exercises that are most appropriate for a client.

_____ 3. Fatigue is a signal that the body is not being cared for properly.

_____ 4. The target heart rate range is 70% to 85%.

_____ 5. Your client can maintain her current physical fitness level by doing her regular workout whenever she feels the need.

_____ 6. When starting a workout, you can work the client just as hard as you would when ending the workout.

WORD SEARCH

Find the words related to designing a conditioning program.

```
o q m a r b c r d c i m i x o
u e v u u l h u m a x o a b b
o p v r a m r i g p t d u w j
s p e c i a l i z a t i o n e
j y z r t d m x r c h f y n c
n i t i i c l g u i d i c o t
p q o e m o e q t t m c n i i
k n q e f t d j p y r a e t v
p a d z z a h i b x w t u a e
e o p o o l s c z u g i q v p
m e n i t u o r p a s o e i u
r e l a x a t i o n t n r t m
n o i s s e r g o r p i f o r
j y t i s n e t n i i s o m a
c o o l d o w n u f t w q n w
```

capacity
cool down
duration
frequency
intensity
mode
modification
motivation
objective
periodization
progression
relaxation
routine
safety
specialization
target zone
warm-up

Chapter 9: Emergency Preparedness and Assessment

Assignment Sheet

Grade _____   Name _____

INTRODUCTION

Preparing for an emergency situation is one of the most essential skills you can learn. A proper response to an emergency situation requires planning and practice *before* the emergency occurs. Establishing a feasible, written Emergency Action Plan, and becoming competent in the ability to perform primary and secondary surveys are essential to emergency preparation.

All assessments (primary, secondary, and isolated injury) are done in accordance with HOPS principles (history, observation, palpation, and stress tests). Each of these is discussed in detail within the chapter. Although emergency training can be intimidating, after reading this chapter you should have a better understanding of how to be prepared for an emergency when one does occur.

SHORT ANSWER

Briefly describe the importance of having good observational skills. Feel free to add examples from the book.

TRUE/FALSE

_____ 1. Establishing and implementing an Emergency Action Plan is one of the most import duties an athletic trainer will perform.

_____ 2. If you are in charge of administering first aid, you must immediately determine if the patient is in a life-threatening condition by performing a systematic sideline evaluation called a secondary survey.

_____ 3. You want to look at the patient's face to make sure the patient is breathing, and listen to the mouth for air movement.

_____ 4. A secondary survey is a head-to-toe physical assessment that is done on patients to determine the extent of illness or injury.

FILL IN THE BLANK

1. An examination of the patient to determine the presence of any life-threatening emergencies is called

   _____.

2. The important steps involved in the primary survey are _____, _____,

   and _____.

3. If the airway is not open, you can open it using the _____ maneuver.

4. HOPS stands for _____, _____, _____, and

_____.

MATCHING

Match each item below to a statement or sentence on the right.

_____ 1. Dorsal, or posterior

_____ 2. Distal

_____ 3. Inferior

_____ 4. Lateral

_____ 5. Superior

_____ 6. Transverse plane

_____ 7. Ventral, or anterior

_____ 8. Frontal, or coronal plane

_____ 9. Medial

_____ 10. Midsagittal plane

_____ 11. Proximal

_____ 12. External

_____ 13. Internal

a. Horizontal line that divides the body into top half and bottom half

b. Imaginary line that divides the human body into right and left sides

c. Those parts located near the middle, or center, of the body

d. Those parts located near the outer sides of the body (away from the center)

e. Uses an imaginary line to separate the body into front and back sections

f. Parts located on the front

g. Parts located on the back

h. Body parts that are located above others

i. Body parts or organs that are located below others

j. Indicates that a body part lies distant to the original reference point

k. Body part that is close to the reference point

l. Location outside of, or near the surface of, the body

m. Location inside the body

EMERGENCY ACTION PLAN

Check with one of your local sport teams and evaluate how prepared they are for an emergency.

Paperwork

Check off the items the team has.

- roster of the athletes
- "Acknowledgment of Risk and Informed Consent" form filled out for all athletes, student trainers, managers, and any student on the team
- "Emergency Insurance Information & Consent to Treat" form
- insurance name, policy number, and family physician's number for all athletes, student trainees, managers, and any student on the team
- Physical Form that includes a health history for all athletes, student trainees, managers, and any student on the team

- any "Special Instructions" for all athletes, student trainees, managers, and any student on the team (for example, for an asthmatic athlete, the form would include information about medications, physician's number in case of any questions, and any signs or symptoms to look for)

Establishing the Emergency Action Plan

This needs to be done for after-school time, school time, away-event time, and in the event the student athlete will be participating off campus. Each Emergency Action Plan will change slightly and place responsibilities on various people. For example, if the cross-country team has an asthmatic runner, who runs 5.5 miles, another athlete who runs with her will need to be aware of the signs, symptoms, and Emergency Action Plan that can be engaged as they train.

Fill in the blanks for your team's Emergency Action Plan.

Name	Responsibility
	Attends to the injured athlete and provides immediate first aid.
	Calls the emergency phone number. (Write down which phone will be used; if a cell phone is used, make sure there is a strong signal where you call from.)
	Initiates crowd control and moves nonessential people away from the scene.
	Meets emergency vehicle and takes EMT staff to the injured athlete. (Could be the same person who called; she could meet the emergency vehicles after notifying the first aid provider that the call had been made.)
	Is in charge of having all the forms. Makes contact with the parents or guardian.
	Accompanies injured athlete to the hospital.

Medical Plan for Visiting Team

Fill out the following checklist for the home team to give to the visiting team. Use your school as an example.

Checklist Item	Please Circle One	Please Fill in
Game manager/Athletic director/Administrator		Name(s):
Physician on duty	Yes No	Dr.: Location:
Athletic trainer on duty	Yes No	Name: Location:
Ambulance	Yes No	Location:
First aid provider	Yes No	Name: Location:
First aid kit		Location:
Ice available	Yes No	Location:
Nearest phone		Location: Access to outside line: Long distance if needed for parent or guardian:
Emergency phone number		
Directions to local hospital or sports medicine group	Write here or attach sheet:	
What insurance plan does hospital accept?	List accepted plans here:	
Hospital phone number	( ) -	
Sports medicine group phone number	( ) -	

MORE MATCHING

Match each item below to a statement or sentence on the right.

_____ 1. A bluish tint to the skin and mucous membranes caused by a decrease in oxygen

_____ 2. To exhale; the act of breathing out

_____ 3. To listen

_____ 4. Abbreviation for *pupils equal and react to light*

_____ 5. Inhalation; the act of breathing something into the lungs

_____ 6. How the injury occurred

_____ 7. Head-to-toe physical; an additional assessment of a patient to determine the existence of an injury

_____ 8. Method used to turn a patient with a spinal injury, in which the patient is moved to the side in one motion

_____ 9. State of unconsciousness or deep stupor

_____ 10. Device made to cut off the side tabs to hinge a helmet's face mask back and out of the way

_____ 11. Examination of the patient to determine the presence of any life-threatening emergencies; the initial assessment of airway, breathing, and circulation

_____ 12. Moist

_____ 13. Expanded or stretched

_____ 14. Gray skin color seen in shock patient

_____ 15. Swelling due to excess fluid in the tissue

_____ 16. System of medical evaluation based on history observation palpation tests

_____ 17. Movement of a joint by muscle contraction

_____ 18. Thorough examination of a specific part of the body to determine the extent of injury

_____ 19. Movement of a joint through a range of motion produced by an outside force

_____ 20. Ability to comprehend one's environment regarding time, place, situation, and identity of person

a. PERL

b. Log roll

c. Ashen

d. Active range of motion

e. Secondary survey

f. Inspiration

g. Clammy

h. HOPS

i. Expiration

j. Trainer's Angel

k. Edema

l. Isolated injury assessment

m. Orientation

n. Passive range of motion

o. Auscultate

p. Coma

q. Cyanosis

r. Distended

s. Mechanism of injury

t. Primary survey

MORE TRUE/FALSE

_____ 1. Looking, listening, and feeling have nothing to do with what could be wrong with the patient.

_____ 2. If the person is cool and clammy, then the person may have a heart problem.

_____ 3. The most important duty an athletic trainer may perform is the Emergency Action Plan.

_____ 4. When you go to an away game, it doesn't make any difference if you know other ways to access the field or where another phone is located in case of an emergency.

_____ 5. When you approach an injured athlete, you must not panic and you must stay in charge of the situation, unless someone of higher authority (EMS, paramedic, physician, registered nurse) takes over.

_____ 6. If the athlete shows any kind of paralysis, leave the patient in the position you found the patient in, and protect the head and neck till EMS arrives.

CROSSWORD PUZZLE

Use the clues to complete the crossword puzzle about emergency preparedness and assessment.

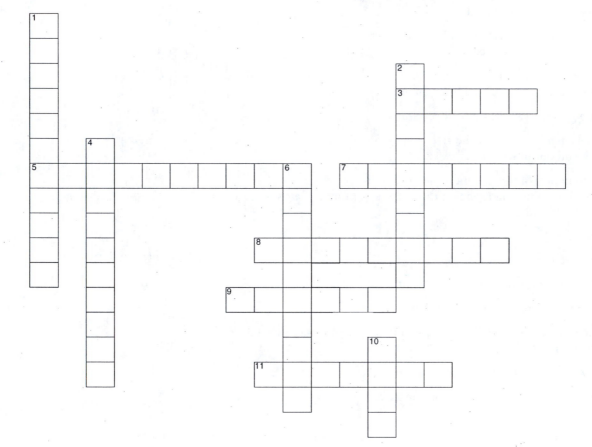

Across
3. Or pale
5. To listen
7. Bluish tint to the skin
8. Expanded or swollen
9. Moist
11. Method used to turn a patient with a spinal injury

Down
1. To inhale
2. Touching
4. Evaluation of a patient's physical condition
6. To exhale
10. State of unconsciousness or deep stupor

Chapter 10: Assembling the First Aid Kits and Equipment Bags

Assignment Sheet

Grade _____   Name _____

INTRODUCTION

This chapter discusses the items needed for each first aid kit, based on the sport being played. Remember that the lists provided in this chapter are suggestions. Budgets and other legal restrictions will greatly influence the contents of many of the kits. These lists are not meant to be memorized, but rather to be used as organizational tools to help you prepare for emergencies. After reading this chapter, you will have a better understanding of how to put together a first aid kit and pack an equipment bag.

SHORT ANSWER

1. An injury report and treatment record should be used for every type of injury that occurs. These forms are important because they document the injuries that have occurred and the treatment that has been provided. In your own words, please explain the three important reasons why injuries and treatments should be recorded.

    a.

    b.

    c.

2. Name the five items that a compact, ready-made first aid kit for any non-ambulance vehicle should contain.

    a.

    b.

    c.

    d.

    e.

3. List the five forms that should be kept as part of your first aid kit.

a.

b.

c.

d.

e.

YOUR OWN FIRST AID KIT

After reading the chapter, make a list of the materials you think you would need in your kit. It is OK to use examples from the book, but it is important that you think of things you would put in your own kit.

TRUE/FALSE

_____ 1. You need at least 100 kits to keep your high school safe.

_____ 2. It is a good idea to have a checklist to make sure you have all of your necessary supplies.

_____ 3. You only need an injury report and a treatment report for yourself.

_____ 4. The personal kit is what you keep with you at home and away games and also during practice.

_____ 5. In football equipment bags, it is good to have extra padding and support that may be needed.

_____ 6. It is very important to rotate the tape in your bag, because otherwise it may become hot and hard to pull off.

_____ 7. In the injury pad bag you never need to get a size larger than XL, because people are never that big.

_____ 8. It is a good idea to meet with the other team's physician to make sure you are familiar with each other's kits.

MATCHING

Match each statement or sentence below to an item on the right.

_____ 1. Report sent to the physician for completion so all interested parties will understand the extent of injury or illnesses

_____ 2. Legal document used to track the course of care for an injured athlete and to evaluate various treatment methods

_____ 3. First aid kit that is kept with you at all times and contains your most essential emergency supplies

_____ 4. First aid kit appropriate for most sports activities

_____ 5. Written report from the athletic trainer to the coach explaining the nature of an athlete's injury or illness, treatment protocols, and suggestions for allowable activities

_____ 6. Items the team physician uses for advanced medical care and treatment that the athletic trainer cannot provide

_____ 7. Instructions for care, given to an athlete or athlete's parents, when a head injury is suspected

_____ 8. Legal document containing information about the nature and treatment of injuries, used to evaluate treatment procedures

a. Basic first aid kit

b. Injury report

c. Coach's injury report

d. Treatment record

e. Head injury and concussion information sheet

f. Personal kit

g. Physician's kit

h. Physician's report

CROSSWORD PUZZLE

Use the clues to complete the crossword puzzle on assembling the first aid kits and equipment bags.

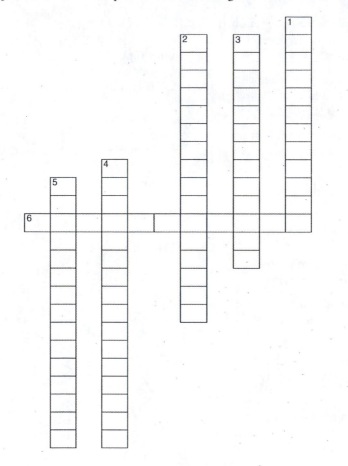

Across

6. First aid kit that is kept with you at all times and that contains your most essential emergency supplies

Down

1. Legal document containing information about the nature and treatment of injuries that is used in the evaluation of treatment procedures
2. A first aid kit that is appropriate for most sports activities
3. Items the team physician uses for advanced medical care and treatment that the athletic trainer cannot provide
4. Is sent with the athlete when he goes to the doctor
5. Legal document used to track the course of care for an injured athlete and to evaluate various treatment methods

Chapter 11: Infection Control

Assignment Sheet

Grade _____   Name _____

INTRODUCTION

The purpose of this chapter is to discuss the importance of preventing injuries from unseen enemies: microorganisms. Signs of infectious and communicable diseases are rarely apparent in everyday encounters. Since you cannot be certain that a patient or an athlete does *not* have a communicable disease such as hepatitis, or is not HIV positive, you must assume that everyone you treat *is* potentially infectious. By washing hands frequently and putting on gloves when treating and evaluating injuries, members of the sports medicine team can significantly reduce the risk of contamination. It is important that you understand the importance of using universal precautions whenever there is the possibility of direct contact with blood or body secretions.

WORD CHOICE

In the following sentences, circle the word in parentheses that correctly completes the sentence.

1. Bacteria are (single-, double-, triple-) celled microorganisms that can destroy blood cells.

2. There is no cure for AIDS, a disease transmitted through blood and sexual contact, which is caused by a (bacteria, virus, monocyte) that attacks the immune system.

3. Hepatitis is a disease that results in the inflammation of the (kidneys, liver, spleen).

4. Contact with blood or body fluids may be hazardous to your health. Thus you should always protect yourself by wearing (lotion, long sleeves, gloves).

5. Washing your hands frequently, wearing gloves and protective clothing when the possibility of exposure to blood or other fluids exists, and keeping your immunizations up-to-date all (prevent the spread of infection, produce a septic environment, make you a cleaner person).

SHORT ANSWER

1. List and briefly explain the six components of the infection cycle.

   a.

   b.

   c.

   d.

   e.

   f.

2. List three of the four guidelines for reducing the risk of puncture wounds from contaminated needles or other sharp objects.

    a.

    b.

    c.

3. Name five types of body fluids that require universal precautions.

    a.

    b.

    c.

    d.

    e.

MATCHING

Match each statement or sentence below to an item on the right.

_____ 1. Guidelines developed by the Centers for Disease Control and Prevention to protect health-care workers from exposure to blood-borne pathogens in body secretions

_____ 2. Acquired immune deficiency syndrome

_____ 3. Sterile, preventing infection

_____ 4. Inflammation of the liver, caused by a virus and spread through contact with infected blood and body fluids; the most common form contracted by health-care workers

_____ 5. Disease-causing microorganism

_____ 6. Removal or destruction of infected material or organisms

_____ 7. Procedure used by health-care workers when assisting with sterile procedures

_____ 8. Inflammation of the liver caused by a virus and spread by the fecal-oral route either from poor handwashing or through contaminated food

a. Pathogen

b. Hepatitis A

c. Hepatitis B

d. Clean technique

e. Sterile technique

f. Universal precautions

g. Aseptic

h. AIDS

TRUE/FALSE

_____ 1. Hepatitis A is spread through blood, blood products, semen, vaginal secretions, and saliva.

_____ 2. Before putting on gloves, one should inspect the gloves for signs of contamination, remove all jewelry, and wash hands and dry the skin well.

_____ 3. An immune system that does not function properly makes a person susceptible to many different kinds of infections, called opportunistic infections.

_____ 4. The infection cycle can be thought of as a chain of events that is given the opportunity to take place when a bacteria, or infectious agent, is present.

_____ 5. It is acceptable to reuse gloves.

_____ 6. It is important that you wash your hands after each patient contact and after removing gloves.

WORD SEARCH

Find and circle the words related to infection control.

```
l  i  m  b  c  a  e  e  a  b  o  m  n  n  g
a  s  e  p  t  i  c  i  i  i  x  e  k  r  l
k  n  d  p  l  e  u  r  a  l  d  t  k  g  o
r  e  i  r  r  a  c  a  t  m  d  s  o  c  v
d  k  c  a  m  n  i  o  t  i  c  y  a  s  e
c  h  a  e  o  a  t  m  u  d  e  s  i  t  s
b  x  l  a  n  i  p  s  o  r  b  e  r  e  c
s  h  a  r  p  c  o  n  t  a  i  n  e  r  s
r  e  s  i  s  t  a  n  c  e  q  u  t  i  y
d  h  e  t  i  s  a  r  a  p  k  m  c  l  n
i  o  p  i  c  l  e  a  n  h  x  m  a  i  o
u  s  s  i  t  i  t  a  p  e  h  i  b  z  v
l  t  i  q  x  f  s  t  c  g  u  z  h  e  i
f  g  s  p  a  t  h  o  g  e  n  k  v  d  a
e  l  i  r  e  t  s  y  a  w  r  i  a  d  l
```

AIDS
airway
amniotic
aseptic
bacteria
carrier
cerebrospinal
clean
fluid
gloves
hepatitis
host
immune system
medical asepsis
parasite
pathogen
pleural
resistance
sharps containers
sterile
sterilized
synovial

Chapter 12: Vital Signs Assessment

Assignment Sheet

Grade _____   Name _____

INTRODUCTION

Measuring vital signs is one of the most important skills a health-care provider will ever learn. The ability to obtain accurate vital-sign measurements is the foundation for proper emergency care. These skills should become second nature to anyone pursuing a career that involves patient care. Continual practice with each of these skills is vital to ensure mastery of the procedures. After reading this chapter, you will have a clearer understanding of how to assess and measure vital signs.

SHORT ANSWER

1. Define *homeostasis*.

2. What is the importance of vital signs?

3. Compare and contrast tachycardia and bradycardia.

4. What are the pulse rates for the following?

    a. Normal pulse rate

    b. Tachycardia pulse rate

    c. Bradycardia pulse rate

    d. Trained athlete pulse rate

5. List five locations the pulse can be felt on the body, and describe each.

    a.

    b.

    c.

d.

e.

6. Name the two different types of temperature scales used to assess a patient's temperature.

a.

b.

7. List five risks associated with excess weight and fat.

a.

b.

c.

d.

e.

MULTIPLE CHOICE

Circle the best answer.

1. The process of bringing oxygen into the body where it can be used by the cells, and expelling carbon dioxide, is called

    a. inspiration

    b. expiration

    c. respiration

    d. inhalation

2. Deep, gasping respirations and air hunger describe

    a. Cheyne-Stokes respiration

    b. dyspnea

    c. apnea

    d. Kussmaul's breathing

3. The normal rate of respiration in populations 15 years of age or older is

    a. 6 to 8 breaths per minute

    b. 15 to 20 breaths per minute

    c. 20 to 25 breaths per minute

    d. 4 to 6 breaths per minute

4. The normal rate of respiration in a well-trained athlete is

    a. 6 to 8 breaths per minute

    b. 15 to 20 breaths per minute

    c. 20 to 25 breaths per minute

    d. 4 to 6 breaths per minute

5. Patients who have difficulty breathing will usually

    a. roll on their side to get more air in and out of the lungs

    b. sit up and lean forward in an effort to breathe easier

    c. stand up and put their arms over their head

    d. sit up and begin to cough

FILL IN THE BLANKS

1. Although blood pressure increases during _____, an exercise program helps _____ blood pressure overall.

2. Low blood pressure may indicate _____, _____, or _____.

3. To get an accurate blood pressure reading, the width of the sphygmomanometer should cover approximately _____ of the patient's upper arm.

4. The body's temperature is regulated by an area in the brain known as the _____.

5. Normal body temperature is _____.

PRACTICING YOUR SKILLS

Now that you have completed the chapter, find a partner and try finding that person's radial and carotid pulse. After you have completed this exercise, practice taking blood pressure measurements with another student in your class.

TRUE/FALSE

_____ 1. Homeostasis is not very important.

_____ 2. The pulse reflects the condition of the patient's circulatory system and cardiac function.

_____ 3. The normal pulse rate for an adult is 60 to 100 beats per minute, with the average heart rate being 70 to 80 beats per minute.

_____ 4. Three main places the heart rate can be found are in the radial pulse, carotid pulse, and the apical pulse.

_____ 5. The brachial artery may be found toward the back of the neck.

_____ 6. Respiration provides the cells of the body with the energy required to perform their specific functions.

_____ 7. The blood pressure of a person always stays the same no matter what the person's weight is or if the person takes steroids or any other type of drug.

_____ 8. To get the patient's temperature readout, you have to make sure the thermometer speculum is inserted into the nose next to the tympanic membrane.

_____ 9. In warm weather glass thermometers cannot be stored in the kits, because if it gets too hot the thermometer will explode.

_____ 10. If a person is overweight, it does not increase the chances of developing cardiovascular disease.

MATCHING

Match each statement or sentence below to an item on the right.

_____ 1. Quantitative measurement of the heartbeat using the fingers to palpate an artery or a stethoscope to listen to the heartbeat

_____ 2. Process of bringing oxygen into the body and expelling carbon dioxide from the body; breathing

_____ 3. State of equilibrium within the body maintained through the adaptation of body systems to changes in either the internal or external environment

_____ 4. Force that the circulating blood exerts against the walls of the arteries

_____ 5. Internal body temperature

_____ 6. Assessments of pulse, respiration, blood pressure, and temperature; body functions essential to life

_____ 7. High blood pressure

_____ 8. Top number in a blood pressure reading

_____ 9. Bottom number in a blood pressure reading

_____ 10. Low blood pressure

_____ 11. Pulse rates lower than 60 beats per minute

_____ 12. Blood vessels that carry blood from the body to the heart

_____ 13. Blood vessels that carry blood away from heart to the rest of the body

a. Blood pressure

b. Pulse

c. Core temperature

d. Respiration

e. Vital signs

f. Homeostasis

g. Diastolic blood pressure

h. Hypertension

i. Hypotension

j. Systolic blood pressure

k. Veins

l. Arteries

m. Bradycardia

LABELING

Label each of the seven pulse points indicated on the following diagram.

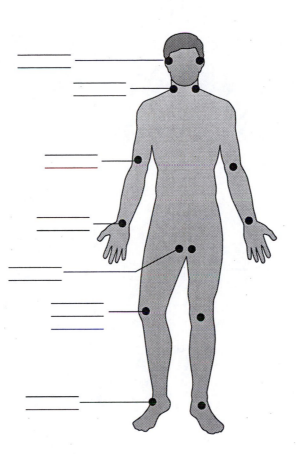

Chapter 13: Basic Life Support

Assignment Sheet

Grade _____   Name _____

INTRODUCTION

The purpose of this chapter is to give you information about basic life support, and the confidence and skills to prepare you to take and pass a certification program in cardiopulmonary resuscitation (CPR). After reading this chapter, you will understand that CPR is done whenever a person's heartbeat and respiration have stopped. It is important that you practice the procedures and skills presented in this chapter. They are vital for any sports medicine professional.

SHORT ANSWER

1. What is the purpose of basic life support?

2. What does *CPR* stand for?

3. List and briefly describe the steps of giving basic life support.

4. In your own words, describe how you would go about removing a foreign body from an unconscious person and a conscious person.

   • unconscious

   • conscious

FILL IN THE BLANKS

1. AED stands for _____.

2. The absence of a heartbeat is called _____.

3. When both _____ and _____ cease, the patient experiences clinical death.

4. After _____ without a _____ or _____, the brain does not receive the oxygen it needs, and the brain cells begin to die.

5. When the brain cells die, it is called _____.

TRUE OR FALSE

_____ 1. If you recognize full arrest and begin CPR an hour later, you can save the patient from biological death.

_____ 2. The best and safest method of opening a child's or adult's airway when a spine injury is not present or suspected is the head-tilt/chin-lift maneuver.

_____ 3. If a spinal injury is suspected, the patient must remain face-down.

_____ 4. If you must begin ventilating for a patient without a mask, obtain a mask as soon as you can.

_____ 5. Trainers and student trainers do not have to be certified in CPR.

_____ 6. A person who is choking usually grabs the throat.

_____ 7. To get food or another substance out of a patient's throat, you can just press on the stomach and the food or other substance will most likely come out.

_____ 8. In the log roll, as long as you are able to roll the patient over, you have no chance of getting hurt.

MATCHING

Match each item below to a statement or sentence on the right.

_____ 1. Log roll

_____ 2. Trachea

_____ 3. AED

_____ 4. Obstructed airway maneuver

_____ 5. Supine

_____ 6. Cardiac arrest

_____ 7. CPR

_____ 8. Back of tongue

_____ 9. Head-tilt, chin-lift maneuver

_____ 10. Xiphoid process

a. Tube of cartilage that extends from the larynx to the bronchial tubes and conducts air into the lungs

b. Position in which the patient is lying flat on the back

c. A lifesaving procedure combining rescue breathing and chest compressions

d. Procedure used to turn a patient over

e. Automated external defibrillator

f. Quick upward thrust against a patient's abdomen

g. Absence of heartbeat

h. Bony tip of the sternum

i. Procedure for opening a blocked airway

j. Epiglottis

CROSSWORD PUZZLE

Complete the following basic life support crossword.

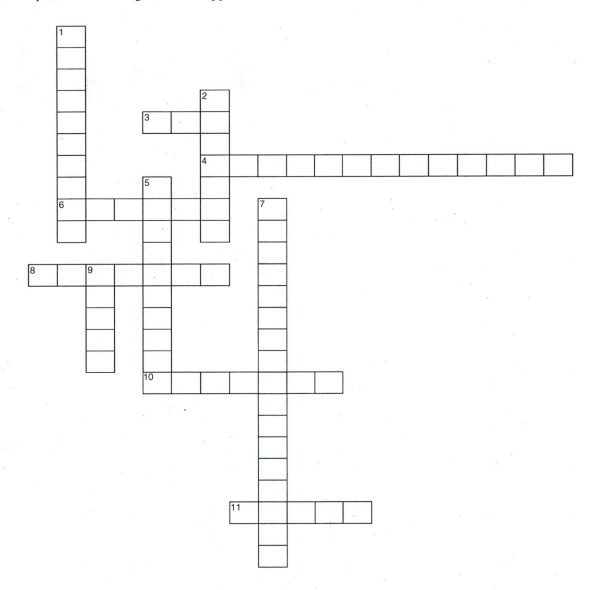

Across

3. Procedure that combines rescue breathing, which supplies oxygen to the lungs, and chest compressions
4. Absence of a heartbeat
6. When a patient is lying on his back
8. Bony tip of the sternum
10. Procedure to turn over a patient lying face-down
11. Acronym for remembering steps to personal safety

Down

1. Respiratory and cardiac arrest is known as _____
2. Also known as the windpipe
5. When the brain cells die
7. When respirations stop
9. Most important sign of circulation

Chapter 14: Injuries to the Tissues

Assignment Sheet

Grade _____   Name _____

INTRODUCTION

A wide variety of injuries can occur during sports and physical fitness activity. Some of the more common injuries involve the tissues, and include cuts and abrasions, contusions, muscle strains, ligament sprains, inflammation of the tendons, joint dislocations, fractures, and injuries to specific organs. Student athletic trainers or fitness instructors must be able to recognize different types of injuries, distinguish between levels of injury severity, and apply appropriate first aid and ongoing treatment to an injured person. When you complete this chapter, you will have a basic understanding of the structure of the human body, the injuries that can occur, and how to treat them.

MATCHING

Match each statement or sentence below to an item on the right.

_____ 1. Structure within the body made up of tissues that allow it to perform a particular function

_____ 2. Open wound, road burn, or rug burn in which the outer layer of skin has been scraped off

_____ 3. Soft tissue injury caused by the penetration of a sharp object

_____ 4. Bubble-like collection of fluid beneath or within the epidermis

_____ 5. Soft tissue injury caused by seepage of blood into tissue; a bruise

_____ 6. Turning, or circular motion, of a body part on its axis

_____ 7. Movement of a body part toward the midline of the body

_____ 8. Movement of a body part away from the midline of the body

_____ 9. Pulled muscle

_____ 10. Inflammation of a tendon

_____ 11. Band of white, fibrous, connective tissue that helps hold bone to bone

a. Blister

b. Rotation

c. Puncture wound

d. Abduction

e. Adduction

f. Organ

g. Abrasion

h. Contusion

i. Ligament

j. Tendonitis

k. Strain

FILL IN THE BLANKS

Cells

1. Cells are made up of a jellylike material known as _____ or _____.

2. Cytoplasm is made of water, carbon, hydrogen, calcium, nitrogen, oxygen, phosphorus, food particles, pigment, and tiny structures called _____.

3. _____ are organelles that release energy and are responsible for the chemical reactions that occur within the cell.

4. _____ are substances contained within the mitochondria and influence the amount of energy released during these chemical reactions.

5. At the center of the cell is the _____, which controls the metabolism, growth, and reproduction of the cell.

6. _____ are found within the nucleus of the cell and contain the _____ that help determine inherited characteristics.

7. The _____ outer covering of the cells is called the _____.

8. Cells reproduce through a process known as cell division. Within the human reproductive organs, this division is called _____.

9. Cell division that occurs elsewhere in the body, such as skin cells producing more skin cells, is called _____.

10. Cells of the same type divide and form _____.

SHORT ANSWER

1. List and describe the four main types of tissue in the human body.

   a.

   b.

   c.

   d.

2. List the eight principles that should be applied when treating any type of wound.

   a.

   b.

   c.

   d.

   e.

   f.

   g.

   h.

3. Compare and contrast a strain and a sprain. Then provide the treatment protocol for each injury.

4. List the four basic parts of the long bones.

   a.

   b.

   c.

   d.

Superficial Injuries

Complete the following chart.

Name of Injury	Immediate Treatment	Follow-up Treatment	Prevention
	Wash area with soap and water, and apply sterile compression dressing to stop bleeding.		Athlete should wear protective clothing and appropriate padding.
Puncture wound		Must be evaluated daily for signs and symptoms of infection.	Make sure the event or practice area is free from nails and other sharp objects.
Incisions	Pull the edges of the wound together using a sterile bandage or butterfly strips.	Change dressing daily.	
Abrasion	Wash wound with antibacterial soap and debride with scrub brush; flush with water; apply dressing to avoid scab forming.		Athletes should wear clothing that protects the skin as much as possible.
	Use compression with a sterile dressing to stop bleeding.	Change dressing daily and watch for signs and symptoms of infection.	Protect the body area with the highest potential for contact.
Calluses	Use a pumice stone on the calluses to file off the thick skin and to stop the problem that is causing friction.		Use of a lubricant, such as Skin-Lube or Vaseline on the area of pressure.
Blisters	Clean area and place a donut pad around the blister to disperse the pressure to the area.	Try to eliminate the source of friction; monitor the affected area for signs of infection.	
Bites	Cleanse thoroughly, and control any bleeding. Bites other than a mosquito bite should be examined by a physician.		Make sure athletes use an insect repellent that will help prevent mosquito bites.
Hematomas		Make sure the patient is seen by a physician.	Make sure all objects near the field of play are padded so that athletes are protected in case they hit the objects.
	Ice, compression, and elevation; apply ice for 20 minutes to constrict the blood vessels, and then remove the ice.	Continue treatment schedule and elevation during waking hours until the swelling has subsided.	Have athletes wear protective pads.

MATCHING

Fractures

Match each statement or sentence below to an item on the right.

_____ 1. Break in a bone

_____ 2. Break in the floor of the orbital socket resulting from a direct blow to the eye

_____ 3. Incomplete break in a long bone shaft in which the bone is also partially bent

_____ 4. Can be caused by repeated stress over time

_____ 5. Break in which one bone fragment becomes embedded in the interior of another bone fragment

_____ 6. Diagonal break that occurs when one end of a bone receives a torsion while the other end remains fixed

_____ 7. Break that occurs across the bone shaft at a right angle to the long axis of the bone

a. Greenstick

b. Blow out

c. Fracture

d. Stress

e. Transverse

f. Impacted

g. Oblique

TRUE/FALSE

_____ 1. Tissue is a collection of similar cells.

_____ 2. Anatomy is the study of the function of the body and how it works.

_____ 3. Cartilage is a fatty tissue.

_____ 4. The ulnar artery is in the leg.

_____ 5. Ice can be used to slow the loss of blood.

_____ 6. A laceration is a jagged tear in the flesh.

_____ 7. A callus is the usually painless thickening in an area with high friction.

_____ 8. To treat a blister, place a pad directly over the blister to decrease the pressure on it.

_____ 9. A hematoma is a swollen, blood-filled area.

_____ 10. Herpes is a viral infection.

MORE MATCHING

Match each statement or sentence below to an item on the right.

_____ 1. A pulled muscle

_____ 2. Fibrous connective tissue around a joint that connects muscle to bone

_____ 3. Stretching or tearing of the ligaments characterized by the inability to move, deformity, and pain

_____ 4. Inflammation of a tendon

_____ 5. Band of white, fibrous, connective tissue that helps hold bone to bone

_____ 6. Crackling or grating sound heard upon movement of a damaged bone or joint

_____ 7. Joint play; motions occurring between the ends of two or more bones that form a joint as it moves through its range of motion

_____ 8. Study of how the body works

_____ 9. Condition in which bone forms in and replaces muscle tissue as a result of trauma

_____ 10. Caused by seepage of blood into tissue; a bruise

_____ 11. Point at which two or more bones meet; a joint

_____ 12. Basic unit of life

_____ 13. Soft tissue injury in which a flap of tissue is torn loose or pulled off completely

_____ 14. Maximum area through which a joint can move

_____ 15. Blood-filled swollen area; a "goose egg" caused by bleeding under the tissue

_____ 16. Reaction that involves the whole body rather than just a part of it

_____ 17. Study of how the body is put together (structure)

_____ 18. Bubble-like collection of fluid beneath or within the epidermis of the skin

_____ 19. Separation of a joint and malposition of an extremity

_____ 20. Inflammation of a bursa

_____ 21. Clean, straight, knifelike cut

_____ 22. Inflammation of the synovial membrane in a joint, characterized by pain, swelling, localized tension, and increased pain with movement

_____ 23. Partial dislocation

_____ 24. Body structure made up of tissues that allow it to perform a particular function

_____ 25. Collection of similar cells and their intercellular substances that work together to perform a particular function

_____ 26. Thickened, usually painless, area of skin caused by friction or pressure

_____ 27. Wound with jagged edges

_____ 28. Open wound, road burn, or rug burn in which the outer layer of skin has been scraped off

_____ 29. Soft tissue injury caused by the penetration of a sharp object

a.   Cell

b.   Myositis ossificans

c.   Articulation

d.   Hematoma

e.   Contusion

f.   Anatomy

g.   Tendon

h.   Strain

i.   Tendonitis

j.   Organ

k.   Systemic reaction

l.   Ligament

m.   Sprain

n.   Physiology

o.   Range of motion

p.   Crepitation

q.   Joint laxity

r.   Tissue

s.   Laceration

t.   Avulsion

u.   Abrasion

v.   Callus

w.   Dislocation

x.   Puncture wound

y.   Subluxation

z.   Blister

aa.   Bursitis

bb.   Synovitis

cc.   Incision

CROSSWORD PUZZLE

Use the clues to complete the crossword puzzle on injuries to the tissues.

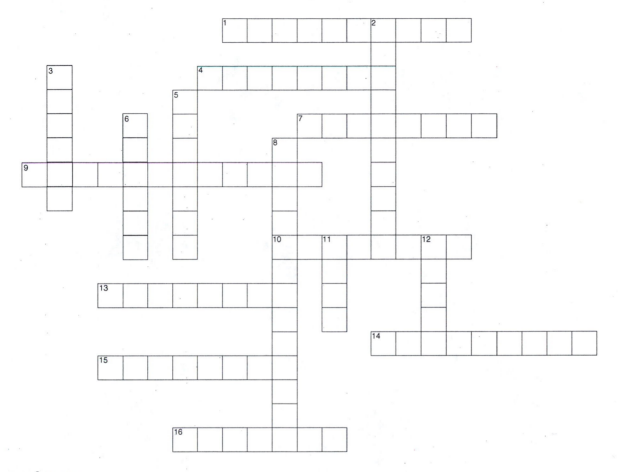

Across
1. Jagged tear in the flesh
4. Loss of tissue
7. Freely movable
9. Tissue fluid
10. A clean, knifelike cut
13. Closed wound
14. Soft tissue injury
15. Open wound
16. Cell division

Down
2. Inflammation of a tendon
3. Voice box
5. Study of how the body was put together
6. A viral infection affecting the face, trunk, and genitals
8. Slightly movable
11. The basic unit of life
12. Structure within the body

Chapter 15: Injuries to the Head and Spine

Assignment Sheet

Grade _____   Name _____

INTRODUCTION

Injuries to the head and neck in sports can be fatal. These injuries must be recognized and treated appropriately to ensure the best possible care and to avoid additional injury. This chapter discusses many of the common sports injuries to the head and spine. After reading this chapter, you will have a better understanding of how to care for and treat the head, neck, and nervous system.

SHORT ANSWER

1. List the two main divisions of the nervous system and the components of each one.

    a.

    b.

2. Describe how you would treat an athlete who is down on the field.

3. List 10 of the 17 possible symptoms of post-concussion syndrome.

4. Use the following box to compare and contrast the three grades of concussion.

Grade 1 (Mild)	Grade 2 (Moderate)	Grade 3 (Severe)
1st Concussion	*1st Concussion*	*1st Concussion*
2nd Concussion	*2nd Concussion*	*2nd Concussion*
3rd Concussion	*3rd Concussion*	

5. Define *kyphosis*.

6. Define *lordosis*.

7. Define *scoliosis*.

8. Compare and contrast spondylolysis and spondylolisthesis.

FILL IN THE BLANKS

1. For each of the following, indicate whether the functions are controlled by the parasympathetic, sympathetic, autonomic, or somatic nervous system.

   a. regulates the balance between the involuntary functions of the body and causes the body to react in emergency situations _____

   b. inhibits salivation _____

   c. contracts bladder muscles _____

   d. constricts bronchi _____

   e. controls skeletal muscles responsible for voluntary movement _____

   f. accelerates heart rate _____

   g. dilates pupils _____

   h. slows heart rate _____

   i. stimulates salivation _____

   j. stimulates the release of epinephrine and norepinephrine _____

2. _____ is the most common injury of the ear in sports activity. It is caused by extreme friction, or by repeated trauma to the ear as occurs in such sports as wrestling and boxing.

3. _____ is an infection of the ear canal. It occurs when moisture is trapped in the _____, or there is a foreign object, an accumulation of earwax, or some other blockage in the ear.

4. A blow to the eye may cause a/an _____. If there is bleeding in the blood vessels around the eye or the temporal regions of the face, _____ may occur.

5. An _____ is a fracture of the bone forming the roof of the eye, caused by a _____ blow to the eye.

6. Inflammation of the membrane lining the eyelid is known as _____.

7. Bleeding within the anterior chamber of the eye is called _____.

8. The result of an infection of the eyelid follicle or the subcutaneous gland is called a/an _____.

9. The septum is the area of _____ between the _____.

10. A nosebleed can also be called _____.

11. One of the most common sports-related injuries to the mouth is to have _____,

_____, or _____.

MATCHING

Match each statement or sentence below to an item on the right.

_____ 1. Sports in which physical contact between players is expected during the normal course of play

_____ 2. Pain that spreads from a central point such as the point of injury

_____ 3. Pain at a location other than the injured organ or site

_____ 4. Severe abnormal discharge of blood

_____ 5. Inability to move

_____ 6. Injury to the brain or spinal cord accompanied by loss of neural function, resulting from a blow to the head or a fall

_____ 7. Individual bone segments of the spine

_____ 8. Nosebleed

_____ 9. Second concussion received before the signs and symptoms of the first concussion have been resolved; life-threatening emergency

_____ 10. Body system composed of the brain and the spinal cord

a. Epistaxis

b. Concussion

c. Vertebrae

d. Second-impact syndrome

e. Central nervous system

f. Paralysis

g. Radiating pain

h. Hemorrhage

i. Contact sports

j. Referred pain

TRUE/FALSE

_____ 1. Constricted pupils are not a result of stimulation of the parasympathetic nervous system.

_____ 2. A person with a second Grade 3 concussion can go back to play after a few days of mild activity.

_____ 3. A person with a Grade 3 concussion does not have any loss of consciousness.

_____ 4. Cauliflower ear is also called hematoma auris.

_____ 5. Bleeding within the anterior chamber of the eye is called hyphema.

_____ 6. Another name for a nosebleed is conchae.

_____ 7. Lordosis is an exaggerated posterior convex curvature of the thoracic spine.

_____ 8. Most back sprains affect the tendons of the facet joints.

_____ 9. Intervertebral disc herniation is a disc that is deteriorated to the point that it pushes against a nerve.

_____ 10. *Spondllidthesis* is spelled correctly.

LABELING

Label each of the brain parts indicated on the following diagram.

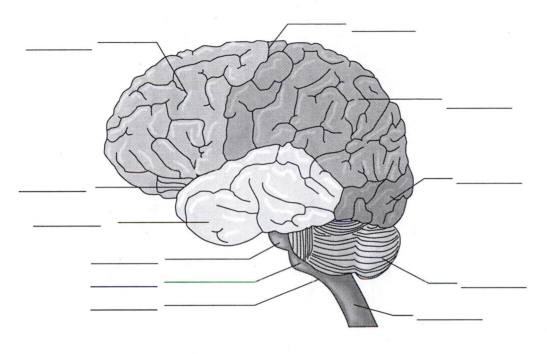

Chapter 16: Injuries to the Upper Extremities

Assignment Sheet

Grade _____   Name _____

INTRODUCTION

The main focus of this chapter is how to perform basic upper extremity evaluations, from the shoulder to the fingers. This involves learning about the anatomy of the upper extremities—including the bones, ligaments, muscles, and tendons—and understanding how they all work together. Please keep in mind that many aspects of anatomy can be difficult to memorize, but continual exposure to three-dimensional anatomical models and meticulous review of the text will help everything fall into place. Although much of this chapter focuses on the evaluation or assessment of injuries, the ultimate goal is to prevent the injuries from happening in the first place.

SHORT ANSWER

1. Name the nine anatomical movements of which the shoulder girdle is capable.

    a.

    b.

    c.

    d.

    e.

    f.

    g.

    h.

    i.

2. Name the four main muscles affecting movement of the shoulder girdle.

    a.

    b.

    c.

    d.

3. Name the four muscles (SITS) that protect the glenohumeral joint.

    a.

    b.

    c.

    d.

4. List the test(s) used to evaluate the following injuries.

    Shoulder fracture

    a.

    b.

    Sprain

    a.

    b.

    c.

    d.

    Strain

    a.

    Impingement

    a.

    b.

    Tendonitis

    a.

FILL IN THE BLANKS

1. The bone in the upper portion of the arm is called the _____. At the proximal end, the humerus attaches to the _____.

2. The four muscles protecting the glenohumeral joint are known collectively as the _____.

MATCHING

Match each statement or sentence below to an item on the right.

_____ 1. Lightly tapping the distal aspect of the athlete's involved bone with index finger

_____ 2. Abducting the athlete's arm to 90 degrees, and slowly performing external rotation

_____ 3. Simultaneously applying a downward force to both elbows causing inferior distraction of the humerus

_____ 4. Test that applies a posterior force to the clavicle

_____ 5. Abduction of the arm followed by controlled lowering to assess the possibility of rotator cuff injury

_____ 6. Application of a medial force to the lateral aspect of a joint in an attempt to create a gap in the medial joint line

_____ 7. Application of a lateral force to the medial aspect of a joint in an attempt to create a gap in the lateral joint line

_____ 8. Tingling sensation produced by percussion of the ulnar nerve

a. Sulcus

b. SC sprain test

c. Tinel's

d. Varus

e. Compression

f. Apprehension

g. Drop arm

h. Valgus

TRUE/FALSE

_____ 1. Epicondylitis is the inflammation of a condyle of the humerus and surrounding tissues.

_____ 2. The wrist is made up of nine bones called the carpals.

_____ 3. Articulation is another name for joint, the place where one bone joins another bone.

_____ 4. Fractures of the wrist and hand, such as a Colles' fracture, usually result from direct blows or falls involving an outstretched hand.

_____ 5. Percussion tests and compression tests are examples of tests used to rule out fractures in the shoulder.

WORD SCRAMBLE

Unscramble these words

1. dtisraconi

2. kannsvklom treoncauct

3. pracla nntuel

4. ttoaror fufc

5. elints gisn

ASSESSMENT CHECK-OFF

Use the following chart to record your progress in mastering the different assessments shown in your text. Your instructor will give you instructions on how and when the assessments will be tested.

Name	Date		Date			Comments
Assessment Check-off	**Peer Check-off** Yes	No	**Instructor Check-off** Yes	No	Score	
Shoulder ROM						
Manual muscle tests for the shoulder						
Shoulder fracture tests						
Sulcus test						
Apprehension test						
Acromioclavicular (AC) sprain test						
Sternoclavicular (SC) sprain test						
Drop arm test						
Hawkins-Kennedy test						
Winged scapula test						
Speed's test						
Elbow ROM						
Manual muscle test, elbow						
Valgus stress test						
Varus stress test						
Tinel's sign						
Wrist ROM						
Manual muscle test, wrist						
Phalen's test						
Finger ROM						
Manual muscle test, finger						
Gamekeeper's thumb test						

CROSSWORD PUZZLE

Use the clues to complete the crossword on injuries to the upper extremities.

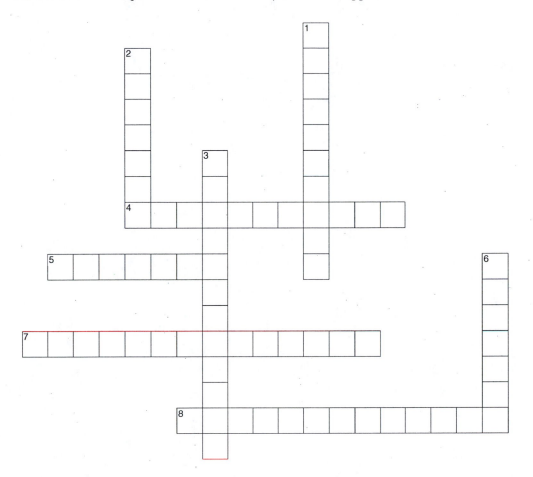

Across

4. Partial dislocation
5. A complete tear of a muscle
7. Tapping a bone to assess the possibility of a fracture
8. Inflammation of the tendon sheath

Down

1. May be used to measure ROM in a joint
2. Wrist is made up of these eight bones
3. Baseball finger
6. Longest and largest bone of the upper extremity

Chapter 17: Injuries to the Chest and Abdomen

Assignment Sheet

Grade _____   Name _____

INTRODUCTION

Unlike injuries to the shoulders or other muscular areas, injuries to the chest and abdomen can be life threatening. Organs in the chest and abdomen move and filter the blood, a function that cannot be changed or interrupted for more than a very short time. After reading this chapter, you will better understand how to prevent and treat injuries to the chest and abdomen.

SHORT ANSWER

1. Name the two major circulatory systems.

   a.

   b.

2. What is coronary circulation?

3. Name the three layers of tissue that make up the heart.

   a.

   b.

   c.

4. What is the function of the erythrocytes?

5. Name the five different types of blood vessels in the body.

   a.

   b.

   c.

   d.

   e.

6. List all the structures in the body that blood travels through, beginning with the two venae cavae.

   a.

   b.

   c.

   d.

   e.

   f.

   g.

   h.

   i.

   j.

   k.

   l.

   m.

7. What are the functions of the lungs?

8. Describe the process of inspiration and expiration.

9. What is the difference between a pneumothorax and a hemothorax?

10. How would you treat an athlete who is hyperventilating after running an 800-meter race?

11. What is flail chest?

FILL IN THE BLANKS

Who Am I?

1. I am the largest of the organs in the chest. _____

2. I protect vital organs and large blood vessels. _____

3. I am connected to the nose, and allow air to pass between the nose and the mouth.

   _____

4. I can be found between the pharynx and the trachea, and am often called the voice box.

   _____

5. I am a collection of dead leukocytes. _____

6. I make up the largest part of the respiratory system. _____

7. I am usually called the "Adam's apple." _____

8. I am the heart's natural pacemaker. _____

9. I am located in the abdomen's left upper quadrant, slightly behind and to the left of the stomach.

   _____

10. I am the largest abdominal organ. _____

11. I am the abdominal organ that produces insulin. _____

MATCHING

Match each statement or sentence listed below to an item on the right.

_____ 1. Blood flow through the muscular tissue of the heart

_____ 2. Two organs of respiration located within the thorax

_____ 3. Protrusion of an organ or part of an organ through the wall of the cavity that normally contains the organ

_____ 4. Upper, or receiving, chambers of the heart

_____ 5. Presence of air in the thorax, due to perforation of the chest wall or visceral pleura

_____ 6. Main artery in the body

_____ 7. Pumping chambers of the heart, located inferior to the atria

_____ 8. Condition that occurs when two or more rib fractures cause the chest wall to become unstable and chest movements are opposite of normal

_____ 9. Tissue that stores energy, insulates, and cushions

_____ 10. Blood within the pleural cavity

_____ 11. Blood vessels that carry oxygen away from the heart to the tissues

_____ 12. Condition that occurs due to inadequate blood flow to the body, which causes very low blood pressure, lack of urine, and other disorders

_____ 13. Flow of oxygen-depleted blood from the right ventricle to the lungs for reoxygenation, and then to the left atrium of the heart

_____ 14. Organ located in the dorsal cavity that filters blood and produces urine

_____ 15. Prolonged deep, rapid breathing that results in decreased carbon dioxide in the blood

_____ 16. Blood vessels that carry oxygen-depleted blood back to the heart

_____ 17. Flow of oxygen-enriched blood from the left ventricle to the body (except the lungs) and return of oxygen-depleted blood to the heart

_____ 18. Abdominal organ that produces insulin and aids digestion

_____ 19. Microscopic air sacs in the lungs responsible for carbon dioxide and oxygen exchange

a. Hernia

b. Hyperventilation

c. Hemothorax

d. Alveoli

e. Kidney

f. Shock

g. Adipose tissue

h. Pulmonary circulation

i. Lungs

j. Aorta

k. Pancreas

l. Flail chest

m. Arteries

n. Pneumothorax

o. Atria

p. Veins

q. Systemic circulation

r. Coronary circulation

s. Ventricles

TRUE/FALSE

_____ 1. Hernias require no surgery and will eventually go away over time.

_____ 2. The kidneys are part of the digestive system.

_____ 3. The spleen is located in the upper left quadrant, slightly behind and to the left of the stomach.

_____ 4. Referred pain of an injured spleen may be present in the left patella.

_____ 5. Symptoms of a chest contusion are similar to those of a rib fracture.

_____ 6. When an athlete has the "wind knocked out of her," she has suffered a blow to the solar plexus.

_____ 7. The heart has four chambers: two atria and two ventricles.

_____ 8. Another name for the tricuspid valve is the mitral valve.

_____ 9. Red blood cells are called erythrocytes.

_____ 10. The large muscle called the diaphragm separates the thorax and abdominal cavity.

_____ 11. The heart's natural pacemaker is called the sino-atrial node.

_____ 12. The pericardial sac is the thin layer of tissue around the heart.

_____ 13. The systemic circulation system nourishes the heart.

_____ 14. As the blood circulates through the lungs, it receives oxygen from the venules.

_____ 15. Blood circulates through the vascular system every 20 minutes.

_____ 16. The second phase of ventilation is called expiration.

_____ 17. A hemothorax is blood within the kidney, due to an injury to that organ.

WORD SEARCH

Find the words related to the organs of the chest and abdomen.

```
B B F E P I K Z A X L C R L N
I G L R F E M I N I I U B S I
L L A Y H W R Y D M N R F S B
U O I T N E R I E N O R E U O
R T L H M A M T C N E L E S L
E T C R L U S O C A O Y A H G
M I H O Y Y I H T I R N S X O
O S E C S R I D R H O D N Q M
L O S Y L O A E R D O N I B E
G G T T L Q T N E A T R I A H
H W T E S R V J O S C D A C L
G O S P A D G Q L M H O Q X U
E P I G L O T T I S L O Y A L
M U I D R A C I P E C U C M A
E L C I R T N E V N M V P K Q
```

ARTERIOLES
ATRIA
BRONCHIOLES
EPICARDIUM
EPIGLOTTIS
ERYTHROCYTE
FLAIL CHEST
GLOTTIS
HEMOGLOBIN
HEMOTHORAX
HERNIA
KIDNEYS
LARYNX
MYOCARDIUM
PERICARDIAL
PULMONARY
SHOCK
SYSTEMIC
VENTRICLE

Chapter 18: Injuries to the Pelvis and Lower Extremities

Assignment Sheet

Grade _____   Name _____

INTRODUCTION

The lower extremities are particularly vulnerable to sports injuries. Prevention of these injuries presents a challenge to athletic trainers and fitness instructors. After reading this chapter, you should recognize and understand how to treat and prevent injuries of the lower extremities.

ASSESSMENT OF LOWER EXTREMITY INJURIES

Use the following chart to document your progress in assessing lower extremity injuries. Your instructor will tell you how and when you will be evaluated by a peer and by the instructor.

Name	Date		Date			Comments
Assessment of Lower Extremity Injuries	Peer Check-off Yes	No	Instructor Check-off Yes	No	Points Earned	
Hip ROM						
Manual muscle tests for hip						
Knee ROM						
Manual muscle tests for knee						
Valgus stress test for knee						
Varus stress test for knee						
Anterior drawer test						
Posterior drawer test						
Lachman test						
Pivot shift						
McMurray test						
Apley compression						
Patella grind						
Ankle and foot ROM						
Manual muscle test for ankle and foot						
Talar tilt test						
Anterior drawer test for ankle						
Thompson test						

FILL IN THE BLANKS

1. Each lower extremity consists of a _____, _____, _____, _____, and _____.

2. The femur is held in the acetabulum by _____, _____, and _____.

3. The _____ extends from the hip to the knee, providing the skeletal structure of the thigh. At the distal end, the medial and lateral condyles of the femur and the tibia _____ with one another. The distal anterior surface of the femur _____ with the _____.

4. Although the _____ is the largest bone in the body, requiring an extraordinary amount of force to fracture, the _____ is not as well protected.

5. On the posterior thigh, the muscle group known as the _____ extends the hip and _____ the knee. The major anterior thigh muscles are the _____.

Who Am I?

1. My symptoms include point tenderness that increases with pressure on the bottom of the foot. _____

2. I am a very contagious fungal infection of the foot, caused by buildup of moisture and heat inside the shoe. _____

3. I cause swelling, heat, and red skin along the front of the leg, along with numbness and reduced ROM in the ankle. _____

4. I am a genetic predisposition that manifests during adolescence as a result of repeated stress to the patellar tendon. _____

5. I am aggravated by a valgus force and can be injured by a lateral blow to the knee. _____

6. I am not stable when an anterior drawer test of the knee is performed. _____

7. I am easily injured by rotation or twisting of the knee. _____

SHORT ANSWER

1. List the four different types of sprains that can occur in the knee.

   a.

   b.

c.

d.

2. The gluteals consist of what three muscles?

a.

b.

c.

MATCHING

Match each statement or sentence listed below to an item on the right.

_____ 1. Test for hip flexor flexibility

_____ 2. Test for tightness of the IT band

_____ 3. Test for weakness of the hip abductors

_____ 4. Bruise or hematoma in the quadriceps muscle

_____ 5. Stretching or tearing of a ligament

_____ 6. Stretching or tearing of a muscle

_____ 7. Ligament positioned inside the knee capsule that prevents anterior translation of the tibia on the femur

_____ 8. Ligament positioned inside the knee capsule that prevents posterior translation of the tibia on the femur

_____ 9. Most commonly sprained ligament in the knee

_____ 10. Test that stresses the lateral collateral ligament

_____ 11. Test to evaluate the integrity of the ACL

_____ 12. Most common cause of a sprained medial collateral ligament

_____ 13. Test to determine the integrity of the PCL

_____ 14. Test performed to identify meniscal tears

_____ 15. Inflammation or irritation of the tibia at its point of attachment with the patellar tendon

a. Strain

b. Medial collateral ligament (MCL)

c. McMurray's test

d. Lachman test

e. Valgus force

f. Osgood-Schlatter disease

g. Trendelenburg test

h. Anterior cruciate ligament (ACL)

i. Posterior cruciate ligament (PCL)

j. Charley horse

k. Posterior drawer test

l. Sprain

m. Ober's test

n. Varus stress test

o. Thomas test

TRUE/FALSE

_____ 1. The knee is a naturally stable joint.

_____ 2. The sesamoid bone that articulates with the distal end of the femur is called the patella.

_____ 3. The main muscles of the lower leg are the tibialis anterior, gastrocnemius, and soleus.

_____ 4. Pointing the toes upward is considered a plantar flexion.

_____ 5. The anterior knee is stabilized by the quadriceps group, which enables extension of the knee.

_____ 6. Inversion is the most common mechanism of ankle sprain.

_____ 7. Dislocations and subluxations cannot occur in the ankle region.

_____ 8. Abrupt stops and starts can cause Achilles tendon ruptures.

_____ 9. Turf toe is caused by hyperextension of the MP joint.

_____ 10. The ligaments of the medial ankle are much larger than those of the lateral ankle.

_____ 11. There is no treatment for shin splints, so athletes must play through the pain.

_____ 12. Chondromalacia patella is always caused by a traumatic event.

WORD SEARCH

Search for the following words related to the lower extremities.

```
G T F I H S T O V I P S J P R A E T N P
S R V Z M C M U R R A Y S F N W S Q C S
L E U P R P X N U C S I D T R O R U Z R
X A W B W Z M Z E C X H E D F Z O S X C
S E C F N S Y T Y C K R W H S X H R J S
P U I H N E A R E C I N O R H C Y E L H
P O S Y M B L T H O M P S O N T E S T I
R U Q R U A T E R G I L D M D R L O Y N
P J D L A D N C D P K N L Z Y A R U R S
Y H U C U T R T J N I Z V G A M A P J P
N M A W C U A L E R E P I N U B H Q S L
Y A X L C L I T G S E R I I Z J C M T I
B O L I A G R A E C T S T R Z Q S M A N
Q P A L A N L H I M Q Y U T L A X Z L T
E T I M E L G R B S V E E S F J R G A S
E K E S E T D E F I K L D M S W X O R X
Y N R T M A A Z S M E P D A S J M D T X
T M A K U C F P F O U A Y H W F H K I X
Z P O Q L I A N E O T N W O R G N I L G
R X F G G W M D P B O Z X X C N H B T W
```

ACETABULUM
ANTERIOR CRUCIATE
APLEY'S
CHARLEY HORSE
CHRONIC
HAMSTRING
INGROWN TOENAIL
LACHMAN TEST
LIGAMENT
MCMURRAY'S
METATARSUS
PATELLA
PATELLA GRIND
PHALANGES
PIVOT SHIFT
QUADRICEP
SHIN SPLINTS
TALAR TILT
THOMPSON TEST
TRENDELENBURG

Chapter 19: Environmental Conditions

Assignment Sheet

Grade _____   Name _____

INTRODUCTION

Being aware of the impact of environmental conditions and preventing environmental emergencies is as vital as proper emergency recognition and response. At some point, most athletes will have to perform in less-than-ideal weather, so the athletic trainer must always be prepared to ensure the athlete's safety.

SHORT ANSWER

1. List and describe the three ways in which the body cools itself.

    a.

    b.

    c.

2. Explain the difference between hypothermia and frostbite.

3. Use the following box to describe the cause and symptoms of different levels of environmental heat stress.

Level of Heat Stress	Cause	Symptoms
Heat cramps		
Heat exhaustion		
Heat stroke		

FILL IN THE BLANKS

1. The heat-regulating center of the body, known as the _____, lies within the brain.

2. Approximately _____ of total heat loss occurs through the skin.

3. For its various temperature-regulating mechanisms to function properly, the body must be well _____, _____, _____, and kept in good _____ through regular exercise.

4. Exertion leads to _____. This depletes the body of _____, and _____ will result if the fluid is not replaced.

5. Fluids can be replaced by _____ or _____.

6. Dehydration is always a possibility when _____, _____, or _____ is present.

TRUE/FALSE

_____ 1. The loss of 1% or less of the body's weight due to water loss impairs athletic performance and increases the risk of heat-related illnesses.

_____ 2. The rate at which perspiration evaporates is strongly influenced by humidity.

_____ 3. Sunburns are caused by ultraviolet (UV) rays from the sun and can cause skin cancer and premature skin aging.

_____ 4. When the blood temperature rises, the hypothalamus sends signals via nerve impulses to constrict the blood vessels in the skin.

_____ 5. Heat is not an important product of chemical activities constantly taking place inside the body.

Chapter 20: Medical Conditions

Assignment Sheet

Grade _____   Name _____

INTRODUCTION

Trainer preparation for pre-existing medical conditions of a client is vital to the proper response to medical emergencies. Having proper knowledge of signs and symptoms of such conditions as diabetes, asthma, seizure disorders, hypoglycemia and insulin shock, appendicitis, genetic heart conditions, and common viruses helps ensure the athlete's safety. Additionally, written doctor's orders for the treatment of special conditions should be available at all times, whether at practice or at competitions.

SHORT ANSWER

1. Compare and contrast a diabetic coma and insulin shock.

2. What role does insulin play in the body?

3. How might a diabetic's breath smell when there are very high levels of sugar in the blood?

4. What is the main concern when a person is having a grand mal epileptic seizure?

5. Why is good hygiene so important when a virus is present in an athletic setting?

FILL IN THE BLANKS

1. _____ is a disease marked by recurring _____ restriction of the bronchi and bronchioles in the lungs. People who suffer from the disease have lungs that are unusually sensitive to _____ and _____.

2. Symptoms of asthma include _____ and _____.

3. _____ is the term that describes a group of nervous system disorders that involve disturbed rhythms of the electrical impulses that fire throughout the _____, resulting in _____ activity or abnormal activity.

4. Inflammation of the appendix is known as _____.

5. Antibiotics are not used for viruses because _____.

Chapter 21: Taping and Wrapping

Assignment Sheet

Grade _____   Name _____

INTRODUCTION

Taping to prevent and treat injuries is part of the science and the art of athletic training. Proper technique is essential to the effectiveness of a taping job, and practice of these techniques allows the athletic trainer to tape faster, better, and with more finesse. After you have read this chapter and practiced the techniques, you will become proficient in this vital skill.

TAPING TECHNIQUE ASSESSMENT

Use the following chart to document your proficiency at various taping techniques. Your instructor will tell you when and how the evaluations will take place.

Name	Date		Date			Comments
Taping Jobs	**Peer Check-off** Yes	No	**Instructor Check-off** Yes	No	**Points Earned**	
Basic ankle strapping						
Combination ankle taping						
Lower tibia taping						
Turf toe						
Arch taping						
Knee strapping						
Achilles tendon taping						
Elbow taping						
Wrist strapping						
Thumb taping						
Finger taping						

SHORT ANSWER

1. List six possible uses of athletic adhesive tape.

   a.

   b.

   c.

   d.

   e.

   f.

2. Define *prophylactic strapping*.

3. What are three ways to increase the tensile strength of tape?

   a.

   b.

   c.

MATCHING

Match each statement or sentence listed below to an item on the right.

_____ 1. Taping that helps prevent injuries

_____ 2. Cloth portion of athletic tape

_____ 3. Degree to which tape is stretched

_____ 4. Synovial membrane inflammation

_____ 5. Ability of fabric or tape to resist tearing

_____ 6. Point at which tape is initially affixed to patient's body

_____ 7. Protective foam material applied to the skin before adhesive tape is applied

_____ 8. Reduced or obstructed blood circulation

_____ 9. Protrusions of bone

_____ 10. Strips of tape applied from one side of the ankle to the other, passing beneath the heel

_____ 11. Inflammation of a tendon

_____ 12. Wrapping tape around a body part in a continuous strip

_____ 13. Cloth tape backed with adhesive used to prevent or support injuries

_____ 14. The first anchor is taped to the underwrap and the skin

_____ 15. Inside of the body part in anatomical position

a. Underwrap

b. Ischemia

c. Backcloth

d. Tendonitis

e. Anchor strip

f. Athletic tape

g. Tension

h. Circumferential wrapping

i. Synovitis

j. Optimal support

k. Stirrup

l. Prophylactic strapping

m. Medial

n. Tensile strength

o. Bony prominences

TRUE/FALSE

____ 1. Table height is not a factor to consider when thinking about the athlete's and trainer's comfort during taping.

____ 2. All brands of athletic tape have the same quality due to how they are made.

____ 3. Layering, or using successive layers of tape, increases the tension of tape.

____ 4. Underwrap is not needed during taping unless the athlete has shaved legs.

____ 5. The roundup is not a method used in the basic ankle tape job.

____ 6. Crimping the tape at the Achilles tendon will increase the tensile strength of the tape job.

____ 7. Most elbow tape jobs are used to prevent hyperflexion.

WORD SEARCH

Find the words related to taping and wrapping.

```
C S O Z T W H Z P F R P N N Z H X Z X P
U N E Z O D B Z Z I F Q G H E L Y D R
V V V G E K L E O A O J T N B W G E E O
L H T G N E R T S E L I S N E T N V O M
O A K F O A J O S E A I S J B U K D V I
P I E T Q V L D H R B E T O D N U X Z N
H R V G P A M A C C I Z H E P O A Z Y E
T A O Q N P X H H R N X D X E D B E J N
O T I P H A T P U P Z A C K L N F E Y C
L N E C H A L J A D H E S I V E T A P E
C Q R N P Y N A A E O T F R U T G N W S
K F D I S I L I H O G W Y H Z S J Q U T
C V N Y B I M A Y P P A R W R E D N U I
A G B M S E O G T F R B Q B I L T C L R
B H U Z H J G N E I U E X X P L S G M R
W H C C H C Y L U K C W T C P I I T R U
T P S N Y L G X Y I D Y E N X H R D C P
K I N R P W G D M R U A Q E I C W T A E
H E E L L O C K Y E O G X I M A Q L R X
G E D P D U R H M X Z J G S P Z L F Z D
```

ACHILLES TENDON
ADHESIVE TAPE
ANCHOR
ARCH TAPING
BACKCLOTH
HEEL LOCK
INTERPHALANGEAL
ISCHEMIA
PHALANGES
PROMINENCES
PROPHYLATIC
STIRRUP
TENSILE STRENGTH
TENSION
THUMB INJURIES
TURF TOE
UNDERWRAP
WRIST

Chapter 22: Return to Play

Assignment Sheet

Grade _____   Name _____

INTRODUCTION

Returning athletes to action after an injury is a frequent occurrence in the life of an athletic trainer. Although the athletic trainer is able to make this decision on her own for a wide variety of injuries, some injuries are serious enough that a physician's approval must be obtained before the athlete can return to play. After reading this chapter, you will have a clearer understanding of the injuries that require a physician's written permission. This chapter also provides guidelines for determining an athlete's readiness for play when no physician's approval is necessary.

SHORT ANSWER

1. List the four circumstances that would require a physician's consent before an athlete can return to play.

    a.

    b.

    c.

    d.

2. List the five steps involved in making an assessment.

    a.

    b.

    c.

    d.

    e.

3. How would you determine if an athlete is ready to return to play if he has sustained an upper extremity injury?

4. How would you determine if an athlete is ready to return to play if she has sustained a lower extremity injury?

5. How would you determine if an athlete is ready to return to play if he has sustained a back or trunk injury?

MATCHING

Match each statement or sentence below to an item on the right.

_____ 1. Facial expression that reflects discomfort

_____ 2. Coming to terms with the outcome of one's prognosis

_____ 3. Extreme feelings of sadness

_____ 4. Engaging in athletic activity while injured, but in a limited way that prevents an injury from becoming worse

_____ 5. Period in the rehabilitation process in which no significant improvement or progress is made

_____ 6. How the injury occurred

_____ 7. Point at which pain affects performance

_____ 8. Lack of feeling or emotion

_____ 9. Acting in advance to avoid or manage an anticipated difficulty

_____ 10. Mental and emotional ability to perform in competition without undue strain on other aspects of one's life

_____ 11. Psychological or physical methods by which an individual adjusts or adapts to a challenge

_____ 12. Estimate of chance for recovery

_____ 13. Identification of the nature of a disease or condition based on scientific information

_____ 14. Refusal to believe something that is true or real

_____ 15. Frustration or hostility

a. Diagnosis

b. Grimace

c. Apathy

d. Anger

e. Mechanism of injury

f. Psychological fitness

g. Prognosis

h. Denial

i. Proactive

j. Acceptance

k. Restricted participation

l. Plateau

m. Depression

n. Coping mechanisms

o. Pain threshold

TRUE/FALSE

_____ 1. Always palpate the uninvolved side first.

_____ 2. ROM is not important when deciding return-to-play guidelines.

_____ 3. Never try pick up an athlete who has fallen face-down.

_____ 4. An athletic trainer uses a prognosis to identify the nature of an injury.

_____ 5. Family life or conditions at home will have no effect on the athlete's return to play.

_____ 6. The denial stage occurs first in the injury process.

_____ 7. Head and spinal injuries require a physician's written permission before the athlete can return to play.

_____ 8. Taping may enhance an athlete's ability to participate while injured.

_____ 9. An athlete does not need to have full pain-free range of motion to return to a sporting contest.

_____ 10. The pain threshold is the same for all athletes.

CROSSWORD PUZZLE

Use the clues to complete the crossword on return to play.

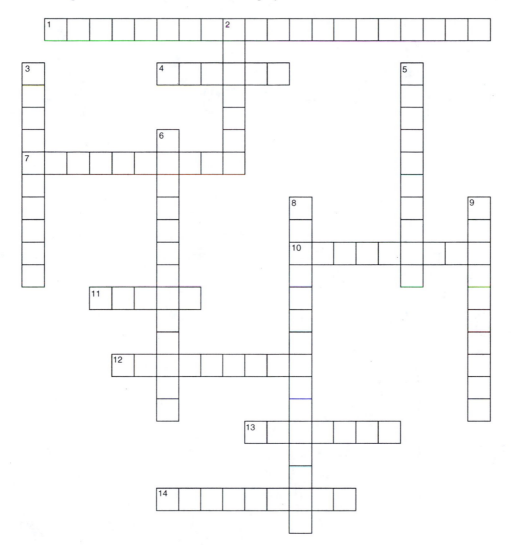

Across

1. Mental and emotional ability to perform in competition without undue strain on other aspects of one's life
4. This coping mechanism usually occurs first
7. Stage in which athletes are able to fully understand and appropriately deal with the extent of their injuries
10. An estimate of a chance for recovery
11. During the _____ stage the athlete is mad at the world
12. Anticipating and preventing as many obstacles to recovery as possible
13. May consist of extended periods during which no increase in strength or ROM is noted
14. Identification of the nature of a disease or condition based on scientific assessment

Down

2. An unspoken indication of pain
3. When this fails, the athlete will experience or return to the anger stage
5. Can result from a variety of life situations—not just injuries
6. The point at which pain affects performance
8. Often emerge in response to stress or change in lifestyle
9. Engaging in athletic activity while injured is this type of participation

Chapter 23: Therapeutic Modalities

Assignment Sheet

Grade _____   Name _____

INTRODUCTION

Therapeutic modalities are methods of applying physical agents to create an optimal environment for healing. They achieve this by increasing or decreasing the patient's bloodflow to a given area following injury or recognition of certain disease processes. If used correctly, these modalities—which include cryotherapy, thermotherapy, and electrical and mechanical, modalities—ease the pain and promote tissue healing. These modalities are the primary tools of rehabilitation. After reading this chapter, you will have been introduced to a wide range of modalities. Some are easy to use safely, but others require formal training or application by a licensed professional.

SHORT ANSWER

1. List the four categories of therapeutic modalities.

   a.

   b.

   c.

   d.

2. Describe the muscle spasm/pain cycle.

3. Name three important factors to consider when selecting a modality to treat an injury or disease process.

   a.

   b.

   c.

4. Compare and contrast thermotherapy and cryotherapy.

5. Name the three phases of sensation experienced by a patient undergoing cryotherapy.

a.

b.

c.

6. List twelve guidelines for electrical modalities.

a.

b.

c.

d.

e.

f.

g.

h.

i.

j.

k.

l.

7. List five guidelines for thermotherapy.

a.

b.

c.

d.

e.

8. List four guidelines for cryotherapy.

a.

b.

c.

d.

9. List the five different types of massage.

    a.

    b.

    c.

    d.

    e.

MATCHING

Match each statement or sentence below to an item on the right.

_____ 1. Treatments that use heat to increase circulation to improve flexibility	a. Conduction
_____ 2. Application of sound waves to a body area to increase circulation	b. Cryotherapy
_____ 3. Distraction or pulling of a body part for rehabilitative purposes	c. Evaporation
_____ 4. Method of heat transfer that takes place through other forms of energy, such as sound, electricity, or chemicals	d. Fluidotherapy
_____ 5. Method of heat transfer by or from its source to the surrounding environment in the form of rays or waves	e. Radiation
_____ 6. Method of heat transfer by direct contact with another medium	f. Ice pack
_____ 7. Method of heat transfer that takes place when a liquid is converted to a gas	g. IFS
_____ 8. Uses ultrasound waves to drive therapeutic agents into body tissues	h. Traction
_____ 9. Interferential stimulation	i. Hydrocollator packs
_____ 10. Moist heat packs	j. Paraffin bath
_____ 11. "Dry" whirlpool	k. Ultrasound
_____ 12. Rehabilitative treatments that use cold to decrease circulation to relieve pain, muscle spasms, inflammation, and edema	l. Phonophoresis
_____ 13. When the arteries and arterioles of an extremity constrict excessively, because of an allergy to cold	m. Thermotherapy
_____ 14. Immersion of a body part in melted wax to increase circulation and flexibility	n. Raynaud's phenomenon
_____ 15. Ice, wrapped in a protective covering, applied to an injury	o. Conversion

TRUE/FALSE

_____ 1. You can apply a cold modality to an open wound without a protective covering.

_____ 2. The most common form of cryotherapy is ice massage.

_____ 3. Vapo-coolant sprays can reduce muscle spasms and increase range of motion, but the effects of such sprays are momentary and superficial.

_____ 4. Typical ice water immersion treatments last 5 to 10 minutes.

_____ 5. Electrical modalities promote healing and reduce pain.

_____ 6. Moist heat packs are a method of heating through conduction.

_____ 7. It is OK to apply heat to the abdomen if there is a possibility that the patient is pregnant.

_____ 8. Heat therapies provide comfort by increasing circulation and decreasing localized pain, edema, muscle spasms, and joint stiffness.

_____ 9. Ultrasound is a low-frequency sound wave that is converted to heat.

_____ 10. Diathermy uses a low-frequency electrical current to heat the body's tissue.

_____ 11. Tapotement is a form of therapeutic massage.

_____ 12. Intermittent compression can be used to help reduce edema.

_____ 13. The temperature of a cold whirlpool is between 55 and 65 degrees Fahrenheit.

_____ 14. Hot whirlpools increase bloodflow.

_____ 15. Paper cups work best for ice massages due to their insulating qualities.

_____ 16. The most common form of cryotherapy is ice packs.

_____ 17. Ice packs are the only form of cryotherapy in which ice is applied directly to the skin.

_____ 18. Moist heat packs decrease circulation.

_____ 19. A paraffin bath can be applied as either a "dip" or "soak."

_____ 20. Never apply any form of cold to anesthetized skin.

WORD SEARCH

Find the words related to therapeutic modalities.

```
Y W H Q C R X S V I A L S A S Y C A T Z
Y T J T H I I P C F O U M S I M O R N P
V S I H A K T E H M X S E C S R N L E P
N A X L V B M E V O A S I U E E D H T N
I T P Q A A N U H P N S A N R H U Y T N
C C T O S D A I S T E O H C O T C F I F
O A E S C D O E F G S T P O H A T J M J
Y S A P V O L M L F A E L H P I I U R A
N G D R A C O A L B A C N P O D O K E V
E P F S S C N L L A O R N A T R N Z T W
T Z E U O A K O A N C U A O O Y E O N G
Q P M A D V O D T N L I R P N P B S I G
T B X I I P W R Q M T B R O O G Z Q I S
H J C V L G A L V A N I C T I V O B M S
T V Q R A S Z Q R O T A L U C O R D Y H
Z S I H T Q R F L U I D O T H E R A P Y
C H Z B I E V A P O R A T I O N L W B U
W T A O O O B W T O K E B I K G U E M Z
R T E H N T W F P W U B S W C P U V T G
H D N U O S A R T L U H A I E T L F K S
```

ANALGESIC
CONDUCTION
DIATHERMY
ELECTRICAL MODALITY
EVAPORATION
FLUIDOTHERAPY
GALVANIC
ICE MASSAGE
ICE PACK
INTERMITTENT
MUSCLE SPASM
PARAFFIN BATH
PHONOPHORESIS
ULTRASOUND
VAPOCOOLANT
VASODILATION
WHIRLPOOL BATH

Chapter 24: Physical Rehabilitation

Assignment Sheet

Grade _____   Name _____

INTRODUCTION

The goal of rehabilitation is to return the patient to a normal life at an effective level of performance. To help patients meet this goal, the rehabilitative environment should reflect a sense of professionalism, motivate the patient, and promote the patient's confidence in a positive outcome. You, along with many other people, contribute to the success of a patient's physical rehabilitation. These people may include the physician, physical therapist, athletic trainer, fitness instructor, physical therapist assistant, physical therapy aide, the patient's family, and others. This chapter introduces you to the process of rehabilitation, including patient assessment and treatment, as well as how information about the patient's progress and treatment is communicated among the team members. After reading this chapter, you will have a better understanding of how to perform assessments, and the importance of patient education throughout every aspect of rehabilitation.

SHORT ANSWER

1. List the different people who make up the rehabilitation team.

   -
   -
   -
   -
   -
   -
   -
   -
   -

2. What four steps should you take to make a patient comfortable?

   a.

   b.

   c.

   d.

3. Describe the first session in any rehabilitation program (include the terms *patient history* and *motivating the patient*).

4. Name the six goals for Phase I of physical rehabilitation.

    a.

    b.

    c.

    d.

    e.

    f.

5. Name the seven goals for Phase II of physical rehabilitation.

    a.

    b.

    c.

    d.

    e.

    f.

    g.

6. Name the six goals for Phase III of physical rehabilitation.

    a.

    b.

    c.

    d.

    e.

    f.

FILL IN THE BLANKS

1. A person's _____ is a visual guide to his body alignment and is assessed on the _____ and _____ planes.

2. Lacking correspondence in shape, proportion, and relative position between opposing body parts is known as _____.

3. Forming right angles to a given plane is known as _____.

4. The instrument used for joint motion measurements is called a _____. _____ is most important when measuring with this instrument.

5. SOAP is an acronym for _____, _____, _____, _____.

TRUE/FALSE

_____ 1. Progress notes written after each treatment session may, at times, follow the SOAP format.

_____ 2. Progress notes will not vary in length and detail.

_____ 3. Plan notes state only your long-term goals with the patient.

_____ 4. The patient history contains facts that are important to the rehabilitation process, as they can affect the design of the rehabilitation plan.

_____ 5. Physical rehabilitation is the process of recovering from an injury.

_____ 6. The abbreviation for "heat pack" is Ht.P.

_____ 7. The first thing performed in a patient's evaluation are functional tests.

_____ 8. Passive ROM is performed before active ROM.

_____ 9. Patient safety, patient needs, patient comfort, and staff conduct are important when creating an optimal environment for healing.

_____ 10. ADL stands for "actions designated for leisure."

_____ 11. Teammates are included in the rehabilitation team.

_____ 12. "Control inflammation" is included in Phase I in any rehabilitation plan.

_____ 13. Phase II of any rehabilitation plan includes remodeling and regrowth.

_____ 14. Nutritional needs do not change simply because of an injury.

_____ 15. Always follow a strict plan in the rehabilitation process.

MORE FILL IN THE BLANKS

Common Abbreviations and Symbols

Write out the names for the symbols and expand the abbreviations below.

1. ACL _____
2. WP _____
3. BP _____
4. US _____
5. PRE _____
6. SLR _____
7. SOB _____
8. DOS _____
9. ↑ _____
10. Δ _____
11. ↓ _____
12. HWP _____
13. FWB _____
14. NWB _____
15. XR _____

MATCHING

Match each statement or sentence below to an item on the right.

____ 1. Reason for performing an action

____ 2. Instrument used to measure the movements and angles created by joints

____ 3. Increase in the posterior protrusion of the thoracic spine

____ 4. Knock-kneed

____ 5. Bowlegged

____ 6. Abbreviation for *whirlpool*

____ 7. Position or alignment of the body

____ 8. Notes on the patient's chart that document patient rehabilitation progress

____ 9. The *P* in *SOAP* notes

____ 10. Devices used to assist injured or weak patients with walking

____ 11. Knees hyperextended

____ 12. Efficient and safe use of the body during activity

____ 13. Rehabilitative treatment that uses physical activity to increase strength and flexibility

____ 14. Abbreviation for *treatment*

____ 15. Forming right angles to a plane

a. Progress notes

b. Exercise modality

c. Posture

d. Body mechanics

e. Crutches

f. Genu recurvatum

g. Goniometer

h. Tx

i. Kyphosis

j. Genu varum

k. Motivation

l. WP

m. Genu valgum

n. Perpendicular

o. Plan

CROSSWORD PUZZLE

Use the following clues to complete the crossword puzzle.

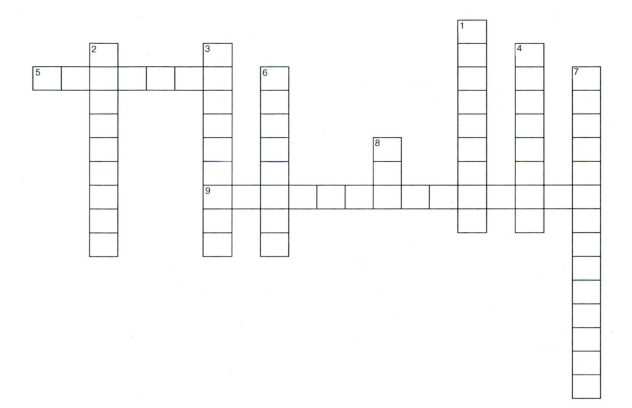

Across

5. Position of alignment of the body
9. Physical _____ is the process of recovering from injury

Down

1. Captain of the rehabilitation team
2. Lacking correspondence in shape, proportion, and relative position
3. Bowlegged
4. Increase in the posterior protrusion of the thoracic curve
6. Devices used to assist injured or weak patients with walking
7. A form that describes the patient's medical history
8. Normal, everyday actions, such as self-care, communication, and mobility skills

Chapter 25: The Selling Point: Promoting Fitness Products and Services

Assignment Sheet

Grade _____   Name _____

INTRODUCTION

Careers in sports medicine require good sales skills. Extensive education, solid experience, and exceptional clinical skills are vital tools of the trade, but they are not enough. The ability to create a positive, capable first impression is a key step to developing a good career in sports medicine. After reading this chapter, you will have the knowledge needed for effective self-promotion.

SHORT ANSWER

1. List the five different types of sales presentations.

   a.

   b.

   c.

   d.

   e.

2. Name some of the items that a professional brochure, Web site, or promotional handout should contain.

   •

   •

   •

   •

   •

   •

   •

   •

   •

   •

FILL IN THE BLANKS

1. Be aware of the importance of personal _____ to a first impression.

2. Be _____. If you have an appointment, arrive at least _____ early. Be _____ and _____ when the time comes.

3. An _____ is a set of steps that you intend to take to achieve your _____.

4. A _____ is an employment plan for the self-employed. Its purpose is to define your _____ and _____ a plan for achieving it.

5. As you create your plan, strive for a healthy balance of _____ and _____ in your life. This requires effective _____ and the ability to _____.

6. Choosing the best sales method depends on your _____, your product or service, your _____, and your _____.

7. Most employment opportunities will require a _____ and a _____.

8. Your _____ should be accompanied by a _____, which serves as a/an _____ and communicates your desire to be considered for a particular position.

9. Promotional materials are not effective unless they are _____, _____, and _____, or at least kept for future reference.

MATCHING

Match each sentence or statement below to an item on the right.

_____ 1. Presentation of one's self or company to buyers through advertising and publicity

_____ 2. Statistical characteristics of given populations used to define business markets

_____ 3. Letter that accompanies a resumé to explain or introduce its contents

_____ 4. Detailed description of the business strategy for an established or start-up business

_____ 5. Detailed description of an individual's strategy for finding employment and advancing in a career

_____ 6. Plan for systematic spending

_____ 7. Immediate and instinctive perception of the truth

_____ 8. Brief written account of personal and professional qualifications and experience prepared by a person applying for a position

_____ 9. Person who organizes, manages, and assumes responsibility for a business

_____ 10. Prompt; not late

_____ 11. Contact friends or colleagues who are knowledgeable in a given area and ask questions

_____ 12. Make doubtful

_____ 13. Self-employment

_____ 14. Achieve the proper balance between career and non-work life

_____ 15. Act of signing or confirming something

a. Resumé

b. Entrepreneur

c. Business plan

d. Demographics

e. Cover letter

f. Intuition

g. Obscure

h. Self-promotion

i. Punctual

j. Employment plan

k. Budget

l. Prioritize

m. Entrepreneurship

n. Networking

o. Endorsement

TRUE/FALSE

_____ 1. It is not smart to put one's company's name or logo on products for promotional reasons.

_____ 2. Having more information on a resumé is always better.

_____ 3. You should write a resumé when you are not in a good mood.

_____ 4. The first impression on a job interview is not always that important as long as you are nice throughout the interview.

_____ 5. Product knowledge, well-developed conversation and memory skills, intuition, a good sense of humor, and the ability to make the client feel comfortable are the keys to successful face-to-face meetings.

_____ 6. Sales presentations are adaptable to a variety of situations.

_____ 7. There are set rules and guidelines that must be strictly followed when making a sale.

_____ 8. Trade shows are excellent opportunities to get to know other professionals in your field and distribute educational materials.

_____ 9. The Internet is not a very good way to sell or buy products.

_____ 10. Good telephone etiquette is not important for telephone interviews; save etiquette for face-to-face interviews.

WORD SEARCH

Find the words related to career and self-promotion.

```
O M P V R T S S S S H A V S S S S I B H
N B A R G U B L N S S T G O E M N S T G
D T S T I U E O L E E C H L N T Z H H W
F V K C D O I N C I Q N F U U V F A L R
R Z Z G U T R N E B K P I I E M U S E R
T G E T O R A I J R R S T S K Y X H M I
G T W M B N E V T O P I L A U T C N U P
D L O F I H R H M I O E O C N B M L V L
O R T F B Y E O G N Z T R M H V A E J R
P P H D C G T N G Y I E Q T W Q N M D M
O X H K Z I T K T G F F B Y N M A I Z E
Z U I P O E E F Q E E E H F L E G T K V
E Y E N E N L M F T A S U W O T E Y Y B
P T P G Z E R Z B A Q N P Z U M M J R A
E N Y G W W E Z B R Q Y R I D S E W Q R
B H G L B I V G I T C J X M N B N K M E
F Q U Q T I O E L S S N P N X D T H Y N
Z B B C S X C O V E R T L Y S S I V S M
V Y E M P L O Y M E N T Q G D R W L B N
U M V U S C I H P A R G O M E D J Z V P
```

BUDGET
BUSINESS
COVER LETTER
DEMOGRAPHICS
EMPLOYMENT
ENTREPRENEUR
FINANCES
HYGIENE
INTUITION
MANAGEMENT
OBSCURE
OVERTLY
PRIORITIZE
PROMOTIONS
PUNCTUAL
RESUMÉ
SELF-PROMOTION
SKILLS
STRATEGY
TIME